I'M SICK OF BEING FAT

How to Lose Weight with Keto

SARAH JANE

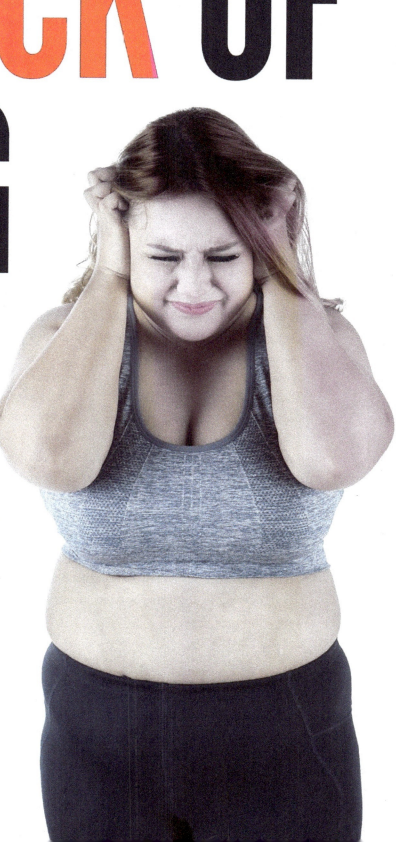

I'm Sick of Being Fat!

How to Lose Weight with Keto

Not for Re-Sale

All rights reserved. All digital products, E-Books, PDF download, resource material, online content and all physical products are subject to copyright protection. Each digital product, E-Book, PDF download and online content is licensed to a single user only. Customers are not allowed to copy, distribute, share and/or transfer the product/s (and/or their associated username/password) they have purchased to any third party or person. Fines of up to $30,000 may apply to person/s found to be infringing our copyright policy.

Legal & Disclaimer

The information contained in this book is not designed to replace or take the place of any form of medicine or professional medical advice. The information in this book has been provided for educational and entertainment purposes only.

All images in this book are licensed and references made to sources of research. The information contained in this book has been compiled from sources deemed reliable, and it is accurate to the best of the Author's knowledge; however, the Author cannot guarantee its accuracy and validity and cannot be held liable for any errors or omissions. Changes are periodically made to this book. You must consult your doctor or get professional medical advice before using any of the suggested remedies, techniques, or information in this book.

Upon using the information contained in this book, you agree to hold harmless the Author from and against any damages, costs, and expenses, including any legal fees potentially resulting from the application of any of the information provided by this guide. This disclaimer applies to any damages or injury caused by the use and application, whether directly or indirectly, of any advice or information presented, whether for breach of contract, tort, negligence, personal injury, criminal intent, or under any other cause of action.

You agree to accept all risks of using the information presented inside this book. You need to consult a professional medical practitioner to ensure you are both able and healthy enough to participate in this program.

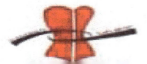

Contents

I'm Sick of Being Fat! 1

    How to Lose Weight with Keto 1

About the Author 12

Introduction 13

Chapter 1: Life is too precious 16

    Hi, I'm Sarah Jane and here is my story… 16

The 5 Myths (Lies) they told us About Losing Weight 22

    1   Eat 5-6 meals per day 22

    2   You can only lose weight by cutting calories and being in a 'Calorie Deficit' 23

    3   You must eat carbohydrates for energy 24

    4   You must do lots of cardio and strenuous exercise to burn fat 25

    5   Eat 'Low-Fat' 26

Understanding the Metabolism 27

Chapter 2: The basics of weight gain 29

    Insulin and Insulin resistance 31

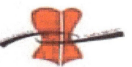

Leptin Resistance 31

Cortisol 36

Thyroid 39

Estrogen 47

Chapter Summary 49

Chapter 3: Preparation 50

Mindset activity 51

Step 1-Goal setting 53

Step 2: Mindset: The Most Important Ingredient 54

10 ways to boost your mindset for weight loss 55

1. Break down large goals into mini- goals 55

2. Surround yourself with a positive network 56

3. Rethink Rewards and Punishments 56

4. Take a Breath 57

5. Patience 57

6. Identify Your 'Trouble Thoughts' 58

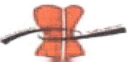

7. Use the scales appropriately 58

8. Be kind to yourself 59

9. Forget the Whole 'Foods Are Good or Bad' Mentality 59

10. Instant motivation boosters 60

Positive Affirmations & Motivation Strategies 61

   Cultivate focus 62

Visualization 62

Step 3: Record Your Starting Point 64

Body Metrics 65

Weight Loss Chart Template 66

Body Measurements Chart Template 66

Step 4: Shopping and meal preparation 72

Chapter 4: Turn your body into a fat melting machine 74

Phase 1: Carb Detox 74

  Protein 78

  Water 79

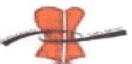

Sauna session 80

Epsom salt bath 81

Natural Fat Burners 83

Ginger 83

Cayenne Pepper 84

Green Tea 84

Nuts 85

Berries 86

Grapefruit 86

Greek Yoghurt 87

Apple Cider Vinegar 88

Green Vegetables (Kale, Spinach and Broccoli) 88

Cinnamon 89

Avocado 90

Chiai Seeds 90

Coconut Oil 91

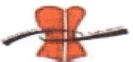

Coffee 91

Garcinia Cambrogia 93

Beta Hydroxy-butyrate (Exogenous Ketone supplement) 93

Green Supplements 94

Metabolism Boosting Recipes 95

Miracle Weight Loss Tea 95

Morning 'Metabolism kick starter' 96

'Keto Mocha Coffee'/a.k.a – 'Bullet proof' coffee 97

Green Smoothie 98

Triple Berry Blast 99

Keto Chocolate Mousse 100

Quick Fat-Burner Salad 101

Café Mocha Smoothie 102

Breakfast Bowl 103

Protein Pancakes 104

Keto -Friendly Mayonnaise 105

Keto Panna Cotta 107

Keto 'Berry' delicious Mousse 108

Keto Coconut Pineapple & lime "Weis Bars" 110

Chapter 5: Daily Meal Plans 111

Day 1 114

DAY 2 115

Day 3 116

Day 4 117

Day 5 118

Day 6 119

Day 7 120

Chapter 6: Ketosis and the Ketogenic diet 121

What is Ketosis? 122

The Basics of a Ketogenic Diet 124

Reducing carbohydrate intake 124

Increasing 'Good Fat' Intake 125

Balancing out salt or sodium intake 125

Don't forget the vegetables 126

Timing 127

Is a Ketogenic Diet Harmful or Dangerous? 128

24 Benefits of the Ketogenic Diet 131

1. Weight Loss 131

2. Anti-aging 132

3. Lowering Blood Sugar (Type 2 Diabetes) 132

4. Cardiovascular Disease and Metabolic Syndrome 133

5. Polycystic Ovary Syndrome (PCOS) 134

6. Brain Function 135

7. Irritable Bowel Syndrome (IBS) 136

8. Increased Mitochondrial Function 136

9. Endurance Performance 137

10. Decreased Pain & Lowered Inflammation 139

11. Stable Energy Levels 139

12. Heartburn 140

13. Fatty Liver Disease 140

14. Migraine Treatment 140

15. Clean Burning Fuel for the Body 141

16. Mood Stabilisation (Autism & Bipolar etc.) 142

17. Easier to Fast 143

18. Parkinson's Disease 143

19. Epilepsy 143

20. Alzheimer's 144

21. Cancer 144

22. Multiple Sclerosis (MS) 146

23. Acne 146

24. General Health and Well-being 147

Chapter 7: How to get started with Keto 148

Transitioning into Keto for Weight Loss 151

Trans Fats 155

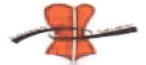

Saturated Fats 156

Unsaturated Fats 156

    Monounsaturated Fats 157

    Polyunsaturated fats 157

Chapter 8: Ketones 159

What are Ketones? 159

Exogenous Ketones 163

What are they and How Can They Help You? 163

What are the Benefits of Exogenous Ketones? 165

So How Will Exogenous Ketones help me to Burn More Fat? 166

Appetite Control: 166

Mitochondrial Biogenesis: 167

Blood Sugar Metabolism: 167

How do Ketones Assist with Brain Function? 168

Improved cognition: 168

Improved mood: 169

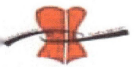

What about my Performance Goals? **169**

    Athletic enhancement: 169

What about Health & Longevity? **171**

    Anti-carcinogenic properties: 171

    Neuroprotection: 171

Ok-So, how do I Get These Exogenous Ketone Supplements? **172**

My Special Thank You to You for Reading This Book…. **173**

Continue with Your Journey **174**

References: **176**

    Journals 178

    Images 179

About the Author

Sarah Jane embodies the frustration many of us have with dieting and trying to lose weight. Sick of the 'yo-yo' dieting, the myths, working hard and not getting results - Sarah then set on a path of creating a program that worked. She was fed up with the conflicting information and just wanted a simple, easy-to-follow plan. Sarah committed to extensive research from doctors, nutritionists and medical journals to collect the relevant knowledge to create what ultimately went into this plan and book.

What makes this book different is Sarah's ability to 'digest' - (pardon the pun) the scientific data and then explain it in such a way that the 'everyday person' can understand! As Sarah has also experienced the struggles with weight and health her motivation and empathy come through the pages. Everything in this book has been tried and tested by the author.

Sarah has a broad experience and background. She is a published author, a qualified trainer/teacher, holds a diploma in nutrition, and a certified keto coach from the great **Dr Eric Berg**. Sarah has over a decade experience as a commercial chef hence the love of food! With this combination she has created some great inclusions in this book such as the 7-day meal plans, recipe suggestions and a holistic approach to a healthy long-term result. Sarah with her self-disclosed medical history of epilepsy, as well as the issues she previously had with her weight, is passionate about finding natural ways to heal the body. Her passion is to help others change their lives through understanding. education, empathy and a touch of fun!

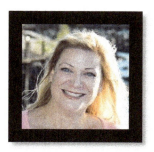

Good luck and happy reading!

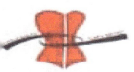

Introduction

Congratulations and well done for investing in this book!

Whatever has got you to this point, sometimes, those experiences may have been painful - instead use them as a blessing –Recognize them as a catalyst for a fresh start and a new you.

You have finally had enough, and you have made the life-changing decision to finally lose the weight and become that version of yourself you have always wanted. Maybe you have medical concerns and/or just don't like what you see in the mirror. Well, now, you have the solution in your hands to get what you have been wanting for so long.

> **TODAY IS THE DAY YOU TAKE YOUR FIRST STEP TOWARDS A HEALTHIER, LEANER AND MORE FABULOUS NEW YOU!**

The definition of insanity is doing the same thing over and over again yet expecting a different result.

If you've tried everything to lose weight and still have not found a permanent solution, then this could be the most valuable message you read all day.

You have tried umpteen things trying to lose the weight. You may even have had success, but then it piles back on PLUS more…. You need to get off this insane merry-go around, once and for all.

But don't give up, all the things you have done to lose weight before haven't worked and it's not your fault, here's why …

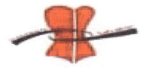

FIRSTLY, losing weight is far more complicated than just calories in versus calories out.
Don't cut back on food trying to lose weight by deprivation.
You wouldn't drive a car with no fuel in the tank, would you?
So why do this to your body?

SECONDLY, you try exercising. I can hear so many groans even at the slightest mention of that word. But the experts tell you that to lose that fat around your tummy and sitting on your hips, you must burn it off. You MUST exercise and lots of it!
So off you go and take your hard-earned cash over to the gym with mirrors floor to ceiling on every wall – you cannot escape your own sorry reflection. Then the personal trainer with the perfect body smoothly signs you up for an expensive membership.
You are very motivated for the first couple of weeks. On you leap onto the treadmill or the elliptical machine and you work on it for hours and hours. Lots of cardio – they said.
But still not having any significant results to show for all your hard work.
You go to a group class and you just can't keep up, it's hard to jump - your joints are sore, every part of your body jiggles and wobbles and you just feel uncomfortable and embarrassed.
So …you give up, but you still must pay for your gym membership.
It's just another thing that's failed.

THIRDLY, you begin to search for something quick. "There must be a 'SECRET'! That's the missing link."
Blinded by the internet hype of Cold Press this, Organic that and drink this Super food blah blah and magically the weight will just disappear.
Sound familiar?

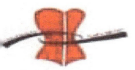

You know it's ridiculous, but you're DESPERATE to get a result after so much effort. You've lost hope. You think it's your fault. Wasted time, effort, money and most importantly your health suffers.

THE GOOD NEWS IS IT DOESN'T HAVE TO BE THIS WAY.

I will show you how you can get your body back without feeling hungry and without feeling like it's another crash diet drag. AND… the results you achieve will be PERMANENT.

Hi, I'm Sarah Jane. I was once sick of being fat and have done something about it and now I want to share my experience and HELP YOU TOO!

I will show you the easy way to balance your hormones and get your body working in sync to rid your excess weight. In fact, on average 1-2Kg weight loss within 5 days* as you rid your body of inflammation. (*Results vary from person to person).

In my book, I will show you exactly how to:
- ➢ How to balance your hormones so that your body no longer holds onto fat.
- ➢ How to re-wire your body to use fats as its source of metabolic energy instead of addictive sugar.
- ➢ How to heal your body from 'dis-ease' and add years back to your life.
- ➢ And much more…

Imagine……

- NO MORE mood swings

- NO MORE of that ugly cellulite.

- NO MORE grabbing fists full of fat from around your hips, tummy and thigh and feeling ashamed of what you have let yourself become.

- NO MORE crash dieting. **After all life is just too precious, isn't it?**

Chapter 1: Life is too precious

Hi, I'm Sarah Jane and here is my story…

Life is precious, and our bodies are the only one we must live our lives in. So, whatever has brought you to the point where you have reached out for help – know that you have come to the right place. This book will start you on your journey to losing that fat. You are not alone in this fight. You've got this!

I have walked the same path as you. In fact, my battles of the bulge started at the age of 16. I got my first ever job working at KFC. It was a real achievement for me and I was so excited. At the same time, it was also nerve-racking trying to learn something new and trying so hard to be good at it. I was going OK in the back-kitchen duties but then they decided to train me on the register. So many buttons on the screen all different colors and so many codes to remember, not only this, but I had to get it right and all the customers were watching me. My heart was beating so fast my hands were literally trembling. I literally felt in a state of panic. Then it all disappeared, I was waking up and looking at my mum and dad and a doctor. The doctor said:

"Hello Sarah, do you know where you are?"

I remember thinking to myself – What a stupid question!

I replied, *"I am at KFC of course!"*

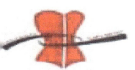

Then I heard laughter.

"What's so funny?"

"Sarah, you're in the hospital. You have had an epileptic seizure. When you have fallen you have cut your back very badly and it will need stitches."

Well, I can honestly say that moment changed my life from then on, it changed my career choices and it also altered my emotions and self-image.

At that age, being diagnosed with a serious medical condition out of the blue was too much to 'digest'; in those years, no one ever talked about being 'depressed'. Clearly looking back, I was.

So, having no real help or outlet, I turned to food to provide the comfort I needed. I would eat and eat and eat, as if trying to push the pain down and to make myself feel better. Then I would feel so guilty having eaten so much. I felt ashamed. Then I just gave up.

My weight increased dramatically. I remember at that age being a lean 48 Kg, and now I was 87Kg and the doctor was telling me:

'You are in the obese category and need to get your weight down"

"What?"

I'm Sick of Being Fat! – Sarah Jane

My dad was never a positive influence in my life (putting that mildly). He would refer to me as being as "*Fat as a bullock*" and "*you will never amount to anything in life*".

I had my first boyfriend at that age – I thought we would marry and as the fairytale goes: 'Live happily ever after....'

However, 2 years down that track, he took me aside one night and said that *"I was too fat, and that he was no longer attracted to me."* That was it.

This was not to be the first time that a man would say those terribly unkind words to me.

So, my journey of trying to lose weight began*

- I tried weight watchers
- Jenny Craig
- Lite 'n easy
- I joined Gloria Marshalls I remember they used to have these wooden lathed rollers and women would sit on them as they rolled around, and it was supposed to move/metabolize the fat. Then they had these beds that would shake and move you up and down -Oh my goodness! What a lot of rubbish they used to 'feed us'.
- I joined gyms and got the leotards and shiny lycra pants, the leg warmers and of course the headband. It was the days of the Jane Fonda workouts and Olivia Newton John – 'Let's get physical!'

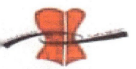

I threw myself into it all. I would have some success, but it inevitably piled back on, so I continued my search for the solution.

- I tried the meal replacement shakes.
- Limits – chocolate biscuits.
- I would eat nothing except pineapples all day – they said apparently pineapple had a special enzyme/ingredient that melted fat.
- I tried the 'cabbage soup diet'.
- I paid hundreds for Garcinia Cambrogia tablets – Celebrity day time presenters recommended them, so it must be true!
- Then it was fat metabolizers and thermogenic supplements. I spent hundreds if not thousands regularly on all kinds of supplements.
- I would go for beauty treatments that smothered you in dead sea salts and then wrap you in thermal foil blankets to heat you up to 'melt away the fat'.
- I had electrical pads connected to a machine and it would move the muscles replicating exercise.
- Increased my meal frequencies to 6 times a day. Only problem was I was now eating more. My 'cheat meals' would become 'cheat months'.
- *Legal Disclaimer – Please note that I am NOT stating that these products/organisation are unsuccessful – I am merely sharing my personal experience and results.*

So, my friend, we have been through it all. **Enough is enough** - this fitness and weight-loss industry has taken my money repeatedly but **failed** to give me results.

I am <u>sick</u> of being <u>**fat.**</u>

I am tired of this insanity! I want a permanent solution – I want to get off this insane *'merry-go around'* once and for all!

That's what has brought me to writing this book. My initial interest was sparked when I heard that the ketogenic diet was helpful for the treatment of epilepsy. I read all the medical journals and the studies. I then started to hear of all the additional benefits that came from following the keto diet especially the fat loss.

I literally read everything I could find, I watched videos, interviews. Searched the web, subscribed to lots of newsletters and now I have put it all together in this book to share with you.

At the time of writing this book, I have begun my transformation. I have successfully lost 3.4 Kg in 3 weeks. So, the evidence in the progress so far is demonstrating that this diet works! Not only showing results just on the scales, but also with a visual comparison with the use of full body photographs side by side. My energy levels have increased. Sleep patterns have improved and the best of all is the brain fog has passed. I have a lot of mental clarity and focus using this ketogenic diet that I never experienced previously. My productivity levels have vastly improved, which means I am getting more out of life. My anxiety levels are decreasing, and my overall mood has shifted upwards. All of which has fueled me to keep going with this new way of life.

Let's stop the old 'diet merry-go-round' - Join me - We will do this together! You are not alone!

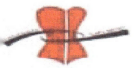

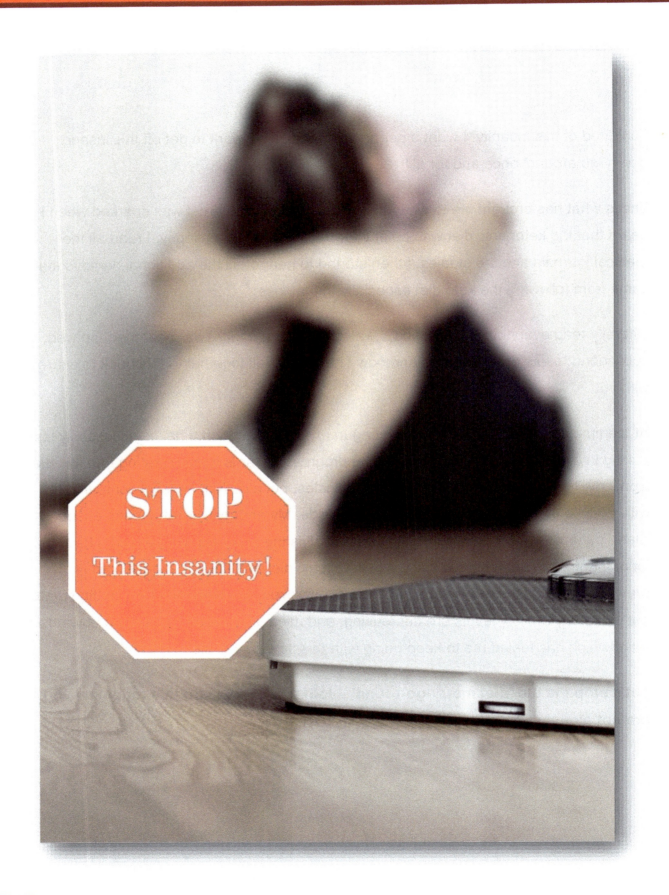

The 5 Myths (Lies) they told us About Losing Weight

1   Eat 5-6 meals per day

We are told that to lose weight we need to "Increase our metabolism". They told us that we must eat 5-6 meals per day so that we don't go into starvation mode '

FALSE! Did you know that medically every time we eat our body naturally releases the hormone 'INSULIN'?

Insulin is a very dominant hormone (It's a fat STORING hormone) that is produced by the pancreas to help reduce blood sugar. Whilst the body is fighting to burn and reduce sugar it CANNOT BURN FAT at the same time.

It can also potentially lead to a condition called 'insulin resistance' which we will discuss later in this book. So, if you want to burn body fat you need to keep insulin low and that means less frequency eating – Don't snack!

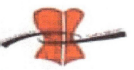

2   You can only lose weight by cutting calories and being in a 'Calorie Deficit'

Losing weight is not as simple as 'calories in and calories out' – otherwise we would be having long term weight issues and epidemic obesity rates worldwide. There is so much more to losing weight than just the calories.

Whilst reducing calories are important and there is some truth to this – it is oversimplified we want to lose weight and we may be in a caloric deficit and we still don't get the results – which is probably because you have a metabolism issue or a hormonal issue – which we will get into later in this book) We cannot continue to keep cutting back more and more calories. Our body needs the basic nutrients to function well and to lose weight. You wouldn't run a car without putting petrol in the tank, would you? So why would you do this to your body?

With the keto diet we focus more on the QUALITY of those calories – what is the macro-nutrients of those calories and are they nourishing your body? Are they helping you to burn fat or to STORE FAT.

Quality of your calories is FAR more important than quantity.

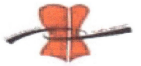

3 You must eat carbohydrates for energy

This is a very long held belief that simply is not true. Our body is very clever in that it can use fat (particularly our own body fat) as an alternative source of energy. This has been used by the body for centuries during times of famine. In the absence of glucose (carbohydrates) the body will turn to its alternative fuel source and that is FATS. Yes, that body fat that sits on your tummy, around your hips and thighs is a source of energy to fuel the body. The way the body does this is using 'ketone bodies' these ketone bodies are produced by the liver and help to break down fats into a useable source of metabolic energy. These ketones can pass through the blood brain barrier and provide glucose energy to the brain and ultimately every cell in your body. Therefore, the body does not actually need carbohydrates it can utilise its own body fat.

I don't know about you but knowing that was one of the most exciting things in weight loss I had heard in decades, and I wanted to KNOW MORE!

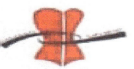

4   You must do lots of cardio and strenuous exercise to burn fat

Your body uses energy just through keeping all of its bodily functions working well in fact this accounts for 70% of our daily metabolic rate. The other 20 % is everyday movements – that leaves only 10% that relates to physical strenuous exercise. Don't; get me wrong exercise does burn calories and is good for us. However, if you have had a LONG-TERM weight issue and you have been exercising and NOT GETTING RESULTS – then wouldn't you say it's; time to shift the focus and find out what is the real cause?

By focussing on getting the body healthy FIRST through nutrition you will give your body the chance to heal and rid itself of the stubborn body fat. Did you also know that most fat -burning is done at night during sleep when your body is in a restorative state? If for example you have high cortisol levels (the stress hormone) you will not be able to get into this restorative state and burn fat. So, all your efforts at the gym are really wasted.

It may be that you have other hormonal issues that is preventing you from losing the weight. This book focusses on nutrition and getting you healthy. It is going to look at the real cause of the weight issue – ONCE we get that RIGHT – THEN we can introduce vigorous exercise programs.

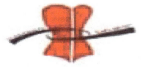

5   Eat 'Low-Fat'

This is another myth that's been in the media for decades. It had everyone eating 'low fat 'foods to lose weight. Yet when manufacturers *'took out the fat'* what they put back in its place was **loaded with sugar and additives**. The damage that the sugar caused us was far GREATER than the damage of fats.

This low-fat strategy was based on a scientist by the name of Ancil Keys. Mr Keys did a study on fat intake in the diet and the link to diseases. His study apparently demonstrated the link between eating high fat and obesity. However, the results of his study were incorrectly released to the media – his study was based on 22 countries yet the result he gave were for 7 countries that he 'cherry-picked' to **manipulate his 'findings'.**

Here is a link if you wish to learn more:

https://deniseminger.com/2011/12/22/the-truth-about-ancel-keys-weve-all-got-it-wrong/

Sugar is far more lethal to our system and is the main cause of weight issues and other health concerns, as we go further into detail in this book I will explain the important function that eating fats has for the body and why you need to keep eating fats but lower your sugar intake.

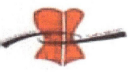

Understanding the Metabolism

Most of us, if not all, believe that if we want to lose weight we have to join a gym, start working out regularly and eventually we will slim down. However, there are 3 main ways our bodies burn calories.

- Resting Metabolism (Basal Metabolic Rate)
- Food Breakdown
- Physical Activity

Basal Metabolic Rate (BMR) refers to the amount of energy the body burns just for its basic functioning. It constitutes most of the energy or calories we burn every day just to sustain living. This includes all your organs such as kidneys, liver, brain and heart. Approximately 70% of our caloric energy is expended here.

The other part of energy expenditure is the thermal effect of food or **Food Breakdown.** It refers to the amount of energy required to break down food in the body. Approximately 10% is expended here.

The third part of energy expenditure is **Physical Activity**. This account varies between 10 to 20 percent of energy use.

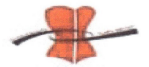

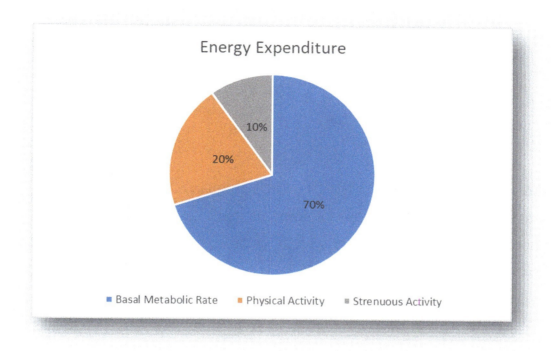

What this means is that to lose weight, we don't have to focus just on strenuous exercise. In fact, nearly 70% of total results is based on nutrition and speeding up the basal metabolism. 20% is everyday movement and only 10% is strenuous activity. Now, hopefully, you will understand why your efforts in the past have failed. It's not you. It's that you have been given the wrong information. In the past, you might have radically changed your eating pattern to something that is completely unsustainable and then added strenuous exercise that your fitness level at that point couldn't cope with. So…. you give up. Well, things are different now; this book will focus on nutrition techniques. The aim is, once you have gained results via this program, you will have the energy and motivation to build up into more active exercise.

Chapter 2: The basics of weight gain

The reasons we HOLD onto fat or BURN fat is dictated in a lot of ways by our hormones. Our hormones are housed in systems made up of a collection of glands that secrete hormones into the circulatory system for various functions. Major glands and organs in this system include; pituitary gland, adrenal glands and the pancreas among others. These glands and hormones are all part of the *endocrine* and neuroendocrine system. All run by the *'Conductor of the Orchestra'* of the body, our brain, via the Hypothalamus. Let's look at some of the big glands that contribute to weight gain and difficulty in losing weight.

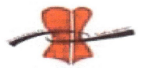

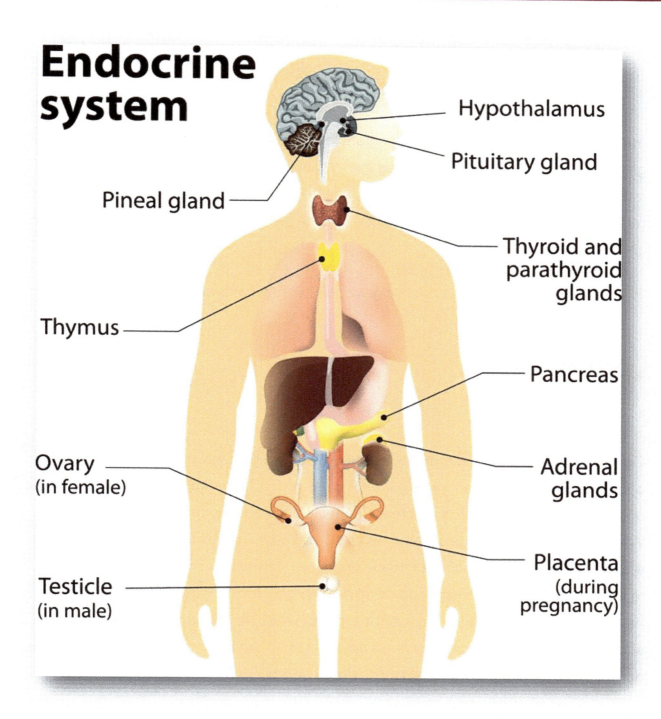

Insulin and Insulin resistance

Insulin is a hormone produced by the pancreas and is responsible for the regulation of glucose(sugar) in the blood as well as the metabolism of fat. The purpose of insulin is to REDUCE blood sugar when you eat/consume sugar or carbohydrates. Insulin is released to get the sugar out of the blood. This sugar is then either:

1. Used immediately for energy.
2. Stored in the muscles/cells as glycogen but most of it will be
3. Stored as FAT!

Leptin Resistance

Our bodies secrete Leptin from the fat cells. When we gain weight, this hormone goes back to tell the brain; *"hey, we've got enough stored fat"*. So, the brain then tells the body to increase metabolism, decrease appetite, increase thyroid and start burning fat. When this hormone was discovered about 15 years ago, it was tested on rats and found they all lost weight. It was like a miracle hormone. However, when it was administered to people, it didn't always work. So, what's going on? Most overweight people tend to have a '**Leptin Resistance**'. So, what happens is that our Leptin goes up as normally it should, but the brain doesn't see it. It's resistant to it. The brain therefore thinks that the body is starving and lowers metabolism, burns less fat.

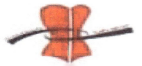

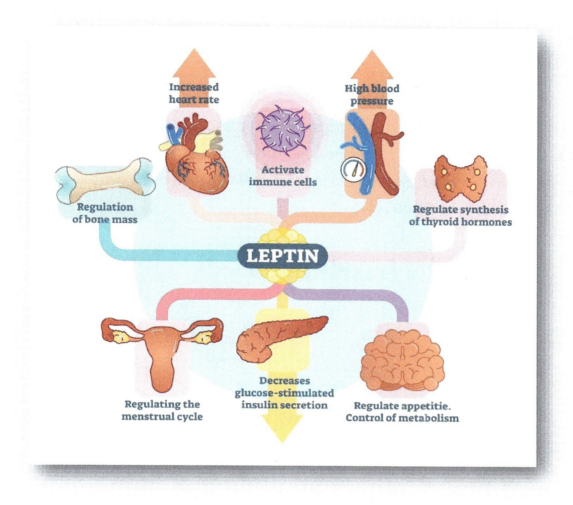

Unless we address this Leptin resistance, we are going to have a very difficult time losing weight. The diagram above shows how Leptin resistance keeps us stuck in a very frustrating cycle. Increased eating and excess calorie intake leads to gaining weight which then leads to an increased amount of fat cells, the higher the fat cells, thus leads to higher Leptin levels. The higher Leptin levels then create Leptin resistance. This Leptin resistance then disrupts the signals transmitted between the brain and the fat cells. But now we have a double whammy – Leptin resistance also pairs up with another hormone – **Ghrelin**

Ghrelin is the hormone that controls appetite that tells us when we are full (Satiety). With this Leptin resistance, our brain scrambles all these messages and tells our body to crave food, and worse still, it does not tell us to stop when we are full. Of course, these important messages then lead to overeating and hence gaining more fat and therefore continuing the vicious cycle.

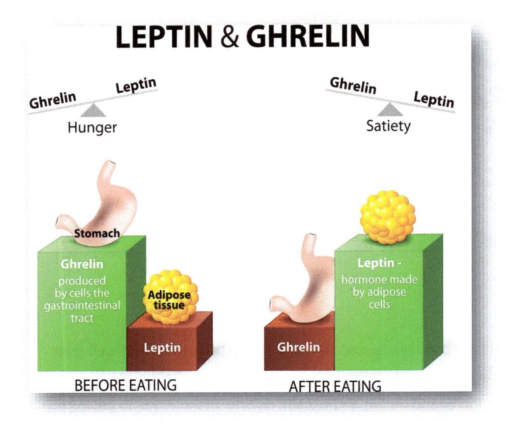

So …how do you diagnose it? Basically, a Leptin level above 12 (see your doctor) indicates that we may have a Leptin resistance. What also happens when people diet significantly and exercise too much, the body will sense stress and lower thyroid levels, hence lowering metabolism.

To show the potency of Leptin resistance factors that control weight, a case study was done at Cambridge University of a child who was of normal weight at birth. The child began to develop morbid obesity very early in life and his parents reported intense increased appetite. The child kept gaining excessive weight and, was weighing 90 pounds by the age of four and was already pre-diabetic. The child had a similarly affected 8-year-old cousin who weighed over 200 pounds. It was later found out that the child lacked the hormone Leptin. Leptin as described earlier is made by fat tissue secreted into the blood where it circulates to the brain to regulate food intake. In the absence of this hormone, human beings and animals eat more. Ultimately, the child was injected with the Leptin made in the lab and he was able to regulate his food intake.

It is now evident that body weight is regulated by a hormonal loop hole of which Leptin is an important component. When we are at a stable weight, our food intake just about equals the energy we produce. We also produce a certain amount of Leptin. If our body weight – specifically the fat tissue in the body – were to fall after going in a diet, the level of Leptin would consequently fall.

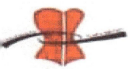

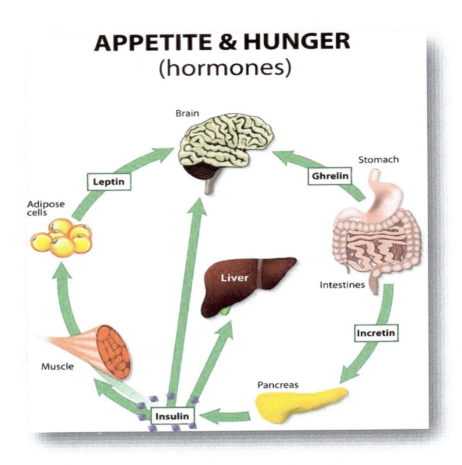

These cravings and appetite can only be resolved when Leptin levels in our bodies are restored to normal levels. Conversely, if you overeat for a period, adipose tissue mass goes up and Leptin level goes up with it, hence suppressing appetite until fat mass and Leptin level return to the starting point. This system sets up a biological response that resists weight change in either direction.

Cortisol

Another hormone that will affect weight issues is the one called Cortisol. Cortisol is a hormone released from the adrenal glands in the kidneys. It is often referred to as "the stress hormone," cortisol levels, rise during tension-filled times. This rise in cortisol triggers the fight or flight response, making the body's fuel sources, such as glucose, ready and available for use. However, if you don't use this energy for a physical response, the body stores the released energy as fat, usually around the abdomen so that it's ready for the next threat. Unfortunately, having high levels of cortisol can turn your overeating into a habit. Because increased levels of the hormone also help cause higher insulin levels, your blood sugar drops and you crave those sugary, fatty foods. So instead of a salad or a banana, you're more likely to reach for cookies or Mac and cheese. That's why they're called 'comfort foods'. Many of us know and recognise now that we can suffer from 'emotional eating'. Eating can be a source of solace to many of us and is an attempt to lower stress. This happens, in part, because the body releases chemicals in response to food that might have a direct calming effect. Fatty and sugary foods are usually the big culprits, because lots of us have such a strong love for them.

Sleep is very important to maintain a healthy weight. When you are not getting enough hours of sleep, normally eight, per night, the hormone Cortisol increases in the blood. This hormone is responsible for storing fat and consistent lack of sleep does increase the amount of fat stored in your body. Also, when you don't get enough sleep, your will-power to make choices decreases.

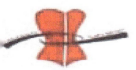

If you are exhausted during the day, that chocolate bar suddenly looks more attractive and you are more inclined to eat it. Getting enough hours of sleep is part of a healthy lifestyle which not only helps with losing weight, but also maintaining a healthy weight. While lack of sleep can lead to weight gain, people who suffer from obesity typically don't get a goodnight's sleep because of sleep apnea. This can cause dangerously low oxygen in the blood causing headaches and fatigue.

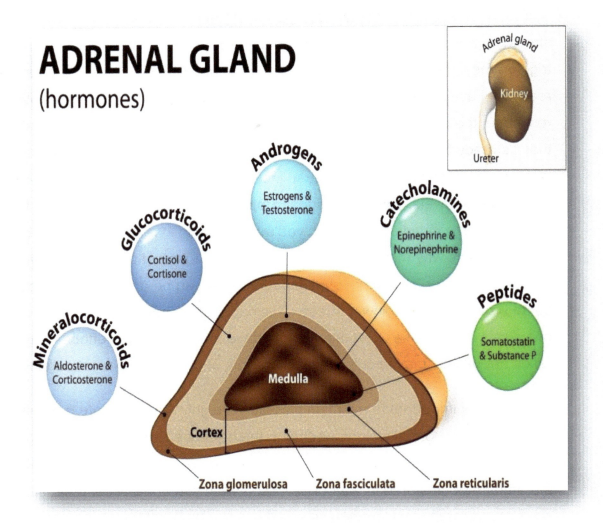

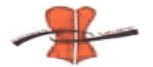

So now that we understand that the hormone cortisol can affect weight gain – what can we DO about it? It's not like we can STOP stress in our lives, can we?

Well, there IS a SOLUTION – I am a warrior for whole foods and natural supplements to heal the body as opposed to any pharmaceutical path if it can be avoided. What I have used and recommend is an 'apoptogenic' herb. What an adaptogen is - is a natural balancer in your body. For example, if your levels are too high, it will lower them and if they are too low, it will raise them. This has been practiced from the Ayurveda medicine. Ayurveda is an Indian health practice thought to be more than 5000 years old. It consists of several disciplines, including aromatherapy, diet, herbal medicine, acupuncture, yoga, massage, meditation and balancing of energies. The word "Ayurveda" is translated from Sanskrit to mean *"the science of life"*.

To assist with balancing the stress hormone Cortisol, I personally have used and achieved great results from an herbal supplement that contains **RHODIOLA.** If you cannot find this herbal supplement, then another effective one is **ASHWAGANDI** – (which also supports the Thyroid – which we will discuss next.) Rhodiola supports exercise endurance and performance and has been traditionally used in Eastern Europe and Asia to relieve fatigue, enhance physical and mental endurance and increase work productivity.

A brand that I highly recommend because it WORKS is:

Stress Ease – Adrenal support – brand is called **Herbs of Gold**

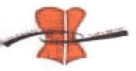

This product contains four herbs supported by the amino acid tyrosine and is formulated to help relieve the stress of study or work – as well as the Rhodiala previously described, it also has Withania, Liquorice and Tyrosine.

Withania is an Ayurvedic tonic used traditionally to restore vitality during debilitation, stress and exhaustion.

Liquorice- has been traditionally used as an adrenal tonic.

Finally, the amino acid, Tyrosine, which is an essential precursor to hormones that regulate stress responses.

If you find that your stress levels are high and suspect Cortisol may be affecting your weight issues – it is well worth trying this natural supplement

Thyroid

Your thyroid is a butterfly-shaped gland situated at the base of the throat, that is an important part of your endocrine or hormone system, it is responsible for maintaining a healthy, balanced metabolism. TSH is the thyroid stimulating hormone secreted by the brain that kicks the thyroid gland to produce hormones. There are two hormones:

T4 (tetraiodothyronine, commonly known as thyroxine) and **T3** (triiodothyronine).

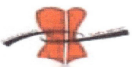

- T4 contains 4 iodine molecules and acts as a *'pro-hormone'* for T3. A 'pro-hormone' means it is then converted in the liver and kidney to the metabolically active T3 hormone. - 80% of your thyroid hormones are actually T4.

- T3 contains 3 iodine molecules and is an active thyroid hormone. T3 is responsible for:
    - Regulation of metabolism
    - Energy production,
    - Body temperature,
    - Body fat, cholesterol,
    - Cognitive function
    - And symptom improvement.

20% of your thyroid hormones are T3, and T3 is 5-7 times stronger than T4. These hormones are responsible for maintaining a healthy, balanced thyroid function.

Thyroid and stress hormones - Your endocrine system contains many glands that produce hormones to help maintain the healthy functioning of other body systems including your reproductive, stress, sugar metabolism and appetite control function. The endocrine system is all linked together, for example, with the release of cortisol during a stressful event it has an impact on the thyroid gland and thyroid hormones

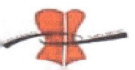

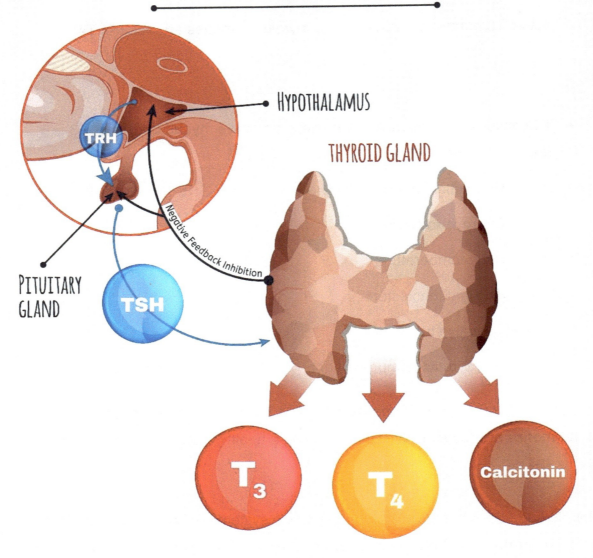

TRH - Thyroid Releasing Hormone
TSH - Thyroid Releasing Hormone
T₃ - Triodothyronine Hormone
T₄ - Thyroxine Hormone

Producing too much thyroid hormone is referred to as hyp**e**rthyroidism. Whilst too little is known as hyp**o**thyroidism. As a result, this slow metabolism will slow the process of burning fat and ultimately lead to weight gain and an inability to lose it despite your efforts.

Other symptoms associated with hypothyroidism are:

- Cold body temperature and poor circulation in the hands and feet
- Fatigue
- Feelings of anxiety and nervousness
- Depression
- Forgetfulness/brain fog
- Muscle and joint pain
- Constipation
- Menstrual irregularities and infertility
- Lack of interest in sex
- Sleeping problems
- Hair starting to thin or fall out
- High cholesterol
- Weight gain

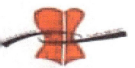

Women are **seven times** more likely than men to develop a thyroid problem and we are particularly vulnerable during times of hormonal change (i.e. after birth, or around the menopause. The cause of thyroid issues can be linked to high cortisol levels or can also be a deficiency in the mineral iodine. The Thyroid Needs Iodine to produce the active hormones T4, T3. Having high estrogen or estrogen dominance can also affect the thyroid as these two hormones compete together and will deplete they thyroid.

So how do we diagnose thyroid issues?

This is done by a simple blood test. However, if you suspect you may have hypothyroidism then you need to request that your doctor do a <u>complete analysis.</u> There are different components of TH that need to be tested. Write this down and take it to your doctor when you ask for your thyroid blood test. All too often, they will test only the TSH– this is insufficient! Without all the tests completed, the TSH may be normal and miss the abnormalities in the T3 and T4. Ultimately, being armed with the full picture will lead to a better solution to the problem.

So, what is the treatment for hypothyroidism?

Your doctor will guide you with medication that is the most appropriate for you. Typically, that will be Thyroxine. However, seeking out natural remedies to heal 'disease', you may be able to support this gland and effectively reduce the need to be on prescription – work with your Doctor on this.

Your food choices are going to be of paramount importance to you. I want you to now AVOID foods that contain gluten, so choose foods such as seafood, walnuts, eggs, spinach, flaxseeds. Look for foods sources that are high in Omega 3 and Omega 6 predominately fatty fish like salmon. Also seek out foods that are particularly high in

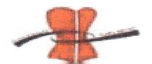

iodine, selenium magnesium and zinc as these are the minerals that the thyroid needs to make the active hormones. In support of the food-based nutritional path, the use of supplements will also be of great benefit to you. There are a few supplements on the market for thyroid issues; however, their efficacy is important to consider so be careful which ones you select.

Another natural herbal supplement you might like to use is ASHWAGANDHA. Ashwagandha, is one of the most powerful herbs in Ayurvedic healing, it has been used since ancient times for a wide variety of conditions and is most well-known for its restorative benefits. In Sanskrit, Ashwagandha means "the smell of a horse," indicating that the herb imparts the vigour and strength of a stallion and has traditionally been prescribed to help people strengthen their immune system after an illness.

Belonging to the same family as the tomato, Ashwagandha is a plump shrub with oval leaves and yellow flowers. It bears red fruit about the size of a raisin. The herb is native to the dry regions of India, Northern Africa, and the Middle East. and today is also grown in more mild climates, including the United States.

Ashwagandha has been used as an apoptogenic herb. An apoptogenic is a natural balancer. What this means is, if your hormone levels are too high, it will lower them and if they are too low it will raise them. It's like an 'auto-pilot' internal mechanism for your hormones!

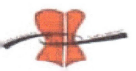

There have been over 200 proven studies on Ashwagandha's ability to:

- **<u>Improve thyroid function</u>**
- **<u>Treat adrenal fatigue</u>** – **balance cortisol**
- Reduce anxiety and depression
- Combat effects of stress
- Increase stamina and endurance
- Prevent and treat cancer
- Reduce brain cell degeneration
- Stabilize blood sugar
- Lower cholesterol
- Boost immunity

In a 20-day study, mice were given ashwagandha and their T3 and T4 levels were analysed along with *'lipid peroxidation'* (anti-oxidant protection). Significant increases in T4 were found which indicates that this herb has a stimulatory effect on a sluggish thyroid. That is great news!

Ashwagandha is available in most good health food stores and may just be the natural solution you are searching for.

Along with Ashwagandha, seek out other ingredients such as:

Iodine helps maintain the body's metabolic rate through the production of thyroid hormone and is an important component of T4 and T3. Iodine is required to produce thyroid hormones and helps to maintain healthy thyroid function.

Selenium is required to produce thyroid hormones and helps maintain healthy thyroid function. Selenium is an important trace mineral needed for the conversion of T4 into the active thyroid hormone T3 via selenium-based enzymes (iodothyronine deiodinase). Deficiency of this enzyme results in reduced conversion of T4 to T3.

Zinc is important for healthy thyroid function as it's needed to produce T4 (thyroxine) via zinc dependant enzymes and a deficiency of these enzymes may affect the production of thyroid hormones.

Tyrosine is required to produce thyroid hormones and helps maintain healthy thyroid function and normal metabolic rate. Tyrosine is also an essential precursor to hormones that regulate stress responses.

As you may have already gathered, there is a link with stress/cortisol and the Thyroid. Some of the natural herbs I have described here can help heal and balance **both** hormonal issues.

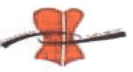

Estrogen

The constant see-sawing of estrogen and progesterone production keeps the reproductive system running. Estrogen plays an important role in the menstrual cycle and pregnancy. It also helps maintain strong bones and may help prevent heart disease.

Are your oestrogen levels out of balance?

A condition called Estrogen dominance' is a significant contributor to weight gain in our older years, particularly when approaching menopause. Spiked estrogen levels can lead to irritability, migraines, painful periods, missed periods, cramps, depression and a raft of reproductive disorders. It is recognised typically by fat deposits around the lower body area: the tummy hips, thighs and buttocks. A person with estrogen dominance will also typically crave carbohydrates.

Another thing that can affect estrogen is what is called 'Endocrine disruptors' these are substances in the environment such as herbicides, pesticides, plastics, hormones that are fed to beef chicken other poultry and GMO foods. Endocrine disruptors 'mimic' estrogen in the body so this will really spike estrogen in the body - this is evidenced by the development of female body parts in a man. This increased estrogen can result in weight gain, fibroids (cysts) on the ovaries, breasts and cancer.

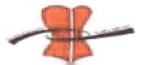

To balance out your estrogen levels you will need to AVOID foods that are Genetically modified (GMO) any ingredients that contains SOY – these are often in protein supplements (Soy Protein Isolate) or diet foods as these are a cheap protein, avoid gluten, wheat, canola and hormone added meats or poultry.

You will need to increase your consumption of 'cruciferous' vegetables – these are your kale, spinach, broccoli, cabbage, cauliflower, Brussel sprouts, radishes etc. These contain high levels of potassium vitamin A and K and also 'Phyto-nutrients' these are natures 'detoxifiers' and have anticarcinogenic properties.

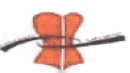

Chapter Summary

Hormones have an enormous effect on how we gain weight and our inability to easily lose the weight. The first step is to identify which of the hormones are causing you the symptoms. Real food, nutrition plans and herbal supplements can help you restore the balance back and get you on your way to shedding the body fat, inflammation and 'disease' in your body. There is finally hope!

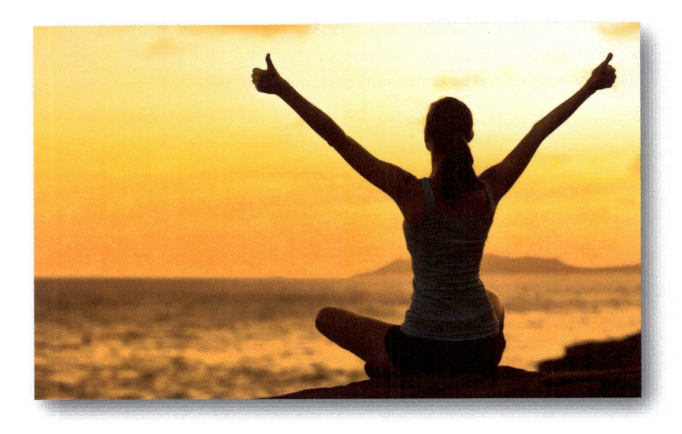

Chapter 3: Preparation

OK – hopefully, now, you are beginning to understand a lot more of what has been going on in your body. Having this knowledge means you are now far more equipped and ready to attack the war on fat! So, let's hit the '**Reset button'** and get ready to fire up your **fat burning!**

One of the issues we faced in the past that have gotten us into this current physical state comes down to what we thought about ourselves. How we respond to situations in our life and our abilities to manage our emotions. So, losing weight is far more than just calories in and calories out. The power of the mind also needs to be given attention. To unravel all of this, we are going to start with your 'WHY'. What is the core reasons why you NEED to make a change and why now? Without coming up with your 'why' when you hit your stumbling blocks – and you will – we all do, your motivations will be the one thing that keeps you on track or even puts you back on track if you fall off. It can be the thing that keeps you moving forward where you need to be.

So, I want you to write down 10 reasons WHY you need to act. Only after you have done this we are going to proceed to set your personal goals; realistic goals. You will then break down these goals into bite-size chunks.

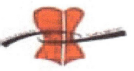

Mindset activity

For this exercise, you are going to use the squares in the table below. Each numbered square represents a year of your life. Take a pen and I want you to color in the age you are now and color in all the ones leading up to it. Then I want you to color in the average age many in your family have lived to. This will be an approximation. Look at the squares that are left blank. These represent the years that you have left in life!

What are you going to do with those precious years that you have left...??

1	2	3	4	5	6	7	8	9	10
11	12	13	14	15	16	17	18	19	20
21	22	23	24	25	26	27	28	29	30
31	32	33	34	35	36	37	38	39	40
41	42	43	44	45	46	47	48	49	50
51	52	53	54	55	56	57	58	59	60
61	62	63	64	65	66	67	68	69	70
71	72	73	74	75	76	77	78	79	80
81	82	83	84	85	86	87	88	89	90
91	92	93	94	95	96	97	98	99	100

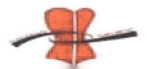

I'm Sick of Being Fat! – Sarah Jane

Next, I want you to really think about WHY you must make a change for your HEALTH, and why you must do it TODAY. Write your reasons in the boxes below.

	I NEED to make changes in my life today because:
1.	
2.	
3.	
4.	
5.	
6.	

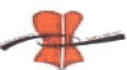

Step 1-Goal setting

Think carefully about what exactly it is you want to achieve and then write out your goals. Goals are a very important part of staying motivated and ensuring you stay on track during your weight loss journey.

To be most effective, a goal needs to be written down and prepared using the S.M.A.R.T principles. SMART is an acronym:

S- *specific*

M- *measurable*

A-*achievable*

R-*realistic*

T-*time framed*

As an example – if you were to say, *"My goal is to lose weight"* a goal such as this is very vague and will not be effective as you don't know when you will achieve that goal. However, a goal created using the SMART principles is a far more powerful strategy.

To get an idea of how to write your goals, follow each of the letters until you get something like this....

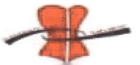

> *"I will lose 20Kg of weight; I will lower my body fat percentage from 45% down to a healthy range of 25%. I will reduce my dress size from a size 20 to a size 14 within 6 months by 31st July".*

A goal written like this will hold you more accountable. It will be a measure of progress and finally it works with the power of the mind. The *'Laws of Attraction'* will work with you to achieve your weight loss aims. When you set your mind a clear intention it will sub-consciously seek out the results you desire.

Step 2: Mindset: The Most Important Ingredient

What we should embrace is the fact that we must get our minds on board. It's no secret that some habits will have to go, but our willingness to embrace change will contribute towards making this journey a true success – PERMANENTLY!

The mindset is perhaps the most important aspect in your weight loss journey. You can't make progress and maintain weight loss if your mind is not on board with the idea. You must ask yourself why you need to lose weight and whether you love yourself enough to keep on moving forward. Set clear goals and then break them down into mini goals so that you don't feel overwhelmed.

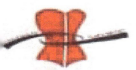

Find an appropriate way to manage your cheat days or cheat episodes because one way or another, it will happen. Get your nutritionist and trainer on board and let them help you work your way through this journey. Gravitate towards positivity by keeping yourself in an emotionally healthy environment. Also, you may want to rethink your rewards and punishment system. Make sure that this is in line with practicing self-care for your body. Always remember, nothing comes easy.

10 ways to boost your mindset for weight loss

1   Break down large goals into mini- goals

Earlier, we described the best method of setting goals. Sometimes, those goals are too large and far away. A good idea is to break the goal down into many smaller more manageable goals. Over which you have full control, they can be as simple as: Did you eat five servings of fruits and veggies today? There's one goal met. What about eight hours of sleep; did you get them in? If so, you can check another goal off your list. Each of the mini goals leads you further towards your goal.

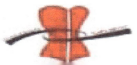

2. Surround yourself with a positive network

Surround yourself with positive people, doing so provides you an encouraging, emotionally healthy environment in which to invest in yourself. Don't be afraid to ask for help or support. There are going to be hard times when you need your network to remind you why you started.

3. Rethink Rewards and Punishments

Keep in mind that making healthy choices is a way of practicing self-care, Food is not a reward, and exercise is not a punishment. They are both ways of caring for your body and helping you feel your best. You deserve both. What this means in terms of rewards is that it doesn't have to be food related, it could be that you achieve a goal and so you go and buy yourself that pair of shoes you've had your eye on. Or you go out on a trip. This will then release you from the physiological trap of emotional eating. You can break the cycle once and for all if you apply this.

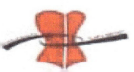

4. Take a Breath

Take a few minutes at the beginning of your workout, or even at the beginning of your day, to slow down and simply focus on the act of breathing. This mindfulness can help you set your intentions, connect with your body and even lower your body's stress response, lie on your back with your legs extended and place one hand on your stomach and one on your chest. Breathe in through your nose for four seconds, hold for four and then exhale through your mouth for four. With each breath, the hand placed on your stomach should be the only one to rise or fall.

5. Patience

Patience is also important when you are losing weight in a healthy and sustainable matter, Plus, if you focus on meeting truly actionable goals, like taking 10,000 steps each day, there's no need to get wrapped up in a timeline of goals ahead. Every 24 hours comes with new successes; focus on those.

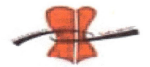

6. Identify Your 'Trouble Thoughts'

Identify the thoughts that get you into trouble and work to stop and change them. Maybe it's your internal dialogue when you consider the mirror. Or those cravings you get for comfort foods when you get stressed. Consciously make them stop by saying 'stop' out loud, it might sound silly, but that simple action will break your chain of thought and allow you the opportunity to introduce a new, healthier one. The best way to do this is to count from one to 100 as many times as you need until the destructive thoughts subside.

7. Use the scales appropriately

While the scale isn't intrinsically bad, a lot of us have learned to associate it with self-destructive thoughts and actions. If that's you, don't even bother stepping on the scale until you get to a place in which the number on the scale doesn't define your worth. Make sure you only use the scale as one of many measuring tools. Remember that changing your body may not always reflect on numbers on the scale. Refer to the previous section on using photographs.

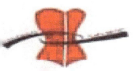

8 Be kind to yourself

Sometimes we are far kinder to others than we are to ourselves. It is fair to say when it comes to ideals of beauty and body image; we are incredibly hard on ourselves. The standards we adopt for ourselves are rather punishing. We would never hold our friends or loved ones to many of those standards. You deserve the same respect and compassion as anyone else; treat yourself kindly.

9 Forget the Whole 'Foods Are Good or Bad' Mentality

Somewhere along the line, we've learned to feel either proud or guilty about every food choice we make. But it's just food, and you shouldn't have to feel guilty about. Let go of the emotional power food may have on you. If you want to have some item that is not on your nutrition plan, then allow yourself a 'cheat' meal – planned and without the guilt and be accountable for your actions.

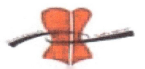

10. Instant motivation boosters

Think about how far you have come. Acknowledge the success you have achieved thus far, and that success will breed success. Perhaps you can keep a journal. Write everything down: When you have a bad day, you can go back and look at a good week and see what you did well. Another clever technique to retrain your brain is to manage your thoughts. Negative self-talk can be very destructive so it's important to stop it immediately. So rather than saying, 'I can't do this', switch it to 'I just haven't achieved it yet'. These words can have a very profound influence on us.

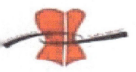

Positive Affirmations & Motivation Strategies

A commonly asked question is; "how we can change these ingrained eating patterns that most of us have had since we were very little?" One of the first things you want to do is to not be over-dependent on willpower to carry you through. A lot of research has suggested that will-power is a finite resource. Think of it like gasoline in the fuel tank in your car. As you run your errands, the gasoline in the fuel tank keeps draining down. Your will-power may be full when you wake up after a good night's rest but depending on what kind of activities you'll do during the day, it will drain a lot or a little. Counting on will-power alone to keep you motivated or keep you on a recipe is itself a 'recipe' for failure.

So, how does one stay motivated? Sustaining motivation over a long term is something that a lot of us have had to struggle with. First, we need to:

Cultivate focus

It may sound rather basic and it is. But here's the thing, we need to revisit our goals periodically, preferably, daily. We need to ask ourselves; "how did I do today?" "How did I do with my goals?" we must have that daily discipline to look and focus on what we're doing and that weekly review. We also need to cultivate a culture of avoiding distractions. It is something that requires us to set boundaries. It takes practice and time to come naturally. When we are focusing on something and really dialing in, it also brings our full presence into that thing, therefore, helping us perform at higher levels. Being positive, that's the key!

Visualization

Visualization is another powerful technique. Close your eyes and see yourself as that new slimmer you. See yourself wearing that great outfit you had waited so long to fit into. Feel how good it feels on your body. Look in the mirror and know you look great. Your loved ones, family and friends all admire how slim and fantastic you now look. Imagine your husband, boyfriend, partner chasing you around the bedroom because he/she can't keep their hands off you!

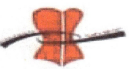

Focus on these mental images whatever they are to you. Intensify the images with bright colors – see the colors of your clothes and your surroundings, add sound to your picture – do you hear your favorite song in the background, or are you on the beach in your sexy bikini listening to the waves rush in and back out and the seagulls. What about the lights – is it dark and romantic with candle light or bright sunshine, whatever is your dream scenario is of you looking the way you have always wanted, zoom in on this picture and ramp up the intensity.

Use your breathing techniques and use the power of the mind to create this reality for you.

Remember you get what you <u>focus on</u> - so focus on what you want!

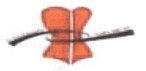

Step 3: Record Your Starting Point

A successful launch of this journey requires you to have certain items with you. Begin by laying some ground work. Purchase a weighing scale if you don't already have one. Getting on the scale and taking body measurements can be quite scary for a lot of us, but you need to know what you're working towards.

Starting my "I'm Sick of Being Fat!" Journey

Insert your start date here:

DAY	MONTH	YEAR
................../	................................../	20....................

Tracking your progress is essential as we have discussed in the previous chapters. Therefore, you will need a system of recording data and your changes. A weight loss chart and a body measurement chart are some proven ways of tabulating your periodic changes. Check out these templates to have an idea of how they should look.

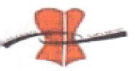

Body Metrics

Height in cm	Weight in lbs. or Kg	Arms	Waist	Stomach	Hips	Chest	Thigh
…………	…………	…………	…………	…………	…………	…………	…………

Take note of the following when making your measurements

- Ensure that the measuring tape is flat and not twisted.
- The tape should not be too tight but should touch your skin all the way around.
- Consistency when taking measurements is important.

Arms: Measure around one arm at the bicep

Waist: Measure around the narrowest part above the hip bones

Stomach: Measure at the navel line

Hips: Measure at the biggest point between your waist and thigh

Chest: Measure at the nipple line or at the biggest point

Thigh: Measure around one leg at the biggest point

Weight Loss Chart Template

Day	Weight	Daily Loss	Day	Weight	Daily Loss
1			11		
2			12		
3			13		
4			14		
5			15		
6			16		
7			17		
8			18		
9			19		
10			20		

Body Measurements Chart Template

Week	Waist	Hips	Thigh	Arm	Stomach	Chest

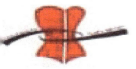

Another powerful technique is using the **visualization transformation technique**.

Get someone to take photographs of you. Choose a plain white background. Clothing must be shorts/briefs for men and ladies a bikini or crop top and briefs.

You will take 3 photographs:

1. Front.
2. Back.
3. Side.

Keep your arms at your sides and no posing.

Here is an example of how to take your 'Before' photographs and then monthly on an on-going basis (progress shots.)

Yes – taking these pictures – stripped down to a bikini is extremely confronting. Nobody ever likes seeing themselves – I certainly didn't. Yet this is an important part of the process. I guarantee that your levels of motivation will increase along with your commitment to reach your goal. You can no longer hide under clothes or make any more excuses.

The need to change for YOU is NOW!

I'm Sick of Being Fat! – Sarah Jane

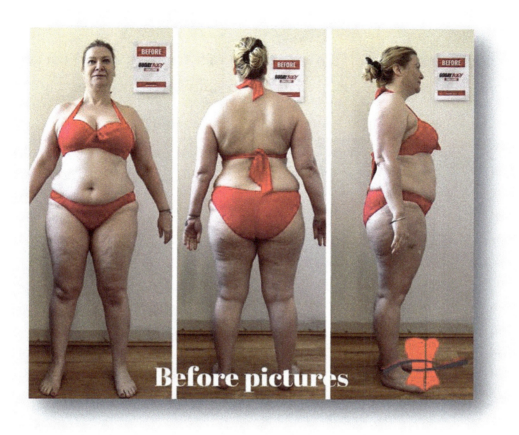

You will repeat this visual method in one month's time. As I said it is <u>extremely confronting</u> - I know because I have felt the same. Sometimes, I even put on weight on the scales despite my efforts, please don't despair – our bodies, particularly women fluctuate with our menstrual cycles, our hormones play havoc and we may have fluid retention. So, don't rely solely on the scales, it's only one method for measuring. Remember there is a big difference between **weight loss** and **fat loss**. We are focusing on reducing body fat not weight loss. So, this technique is very effective in that regard, in fact when you see your photographs you will start to notice physical changes in your own body.

Here is an example:

Here is my original start weight: I am not pleased with it but that's why I am acting - just like you are. It does put me in the medical 'obese' category – such a terribly cruel term.

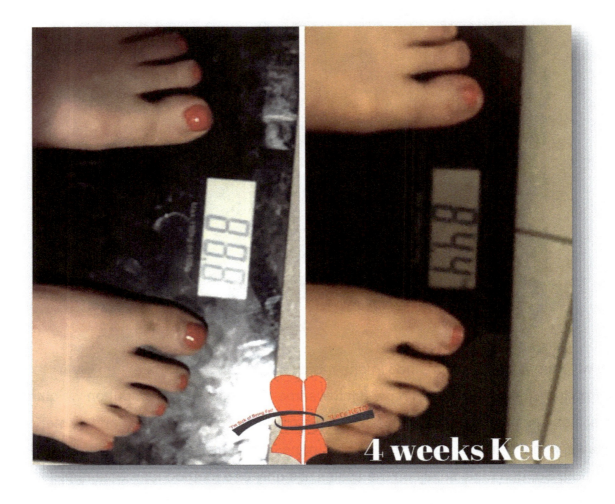

I'm Sick of Being Fat! – Sarah Jane

Now 4.4 Kg weight loss in 4 weeks is quite a good rate of progress but we are the harshest judges of ourselves more so than other people in our lives. So, without taking my pictures I wouldn't really be seeing the changes in my body from the outside.

Here are my body pictures – I have only done mid-section as I don't have anyone to take the picture full length and don't want the photo in the mirror. However, whatever you do, be consistent for comparison sake. I usually take these each week.

This is my real life 4 weeks photo

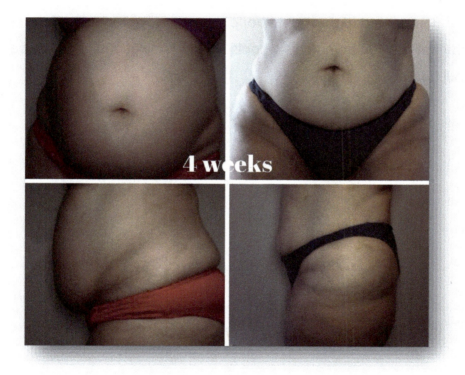

You can see in the first photograph the bloating in my tummy. This was not posed, it is a natural stance. This explains why we feel bloated and tired with little to no energy. Our body is full of toxins and inflammation. Once we get rid our body of inflammatory foods, balance our hormones and eat the right foods, the body will naturally detoxify and get rid of that stubborn fat.

Looking at the 4th week picture, you can see that my tummy has now started to flatten down. What got me even more excited was I started to see my waist taking shape. I look less (to me) like a 'beach balloon' and more like **the hourglass figure I am meant to be** underneath. If I looked even closer, I could even see some lines at the outside length of my abdomen and at the side. I hope you can now understand that 4.4 Kg on the scales may not get you doing cart-wheels – but I know if you see changes in your body – You will be eager to keep going.

Step 4: Shopping and meal preparation

Chicken breast skin off – 1 Kg	Sweet potato x 1 large
Beef steak 300g	Cucumber x 2
Green banana prawns 200g	Coconut oil – organic virgin
Lean Beef strips or beef tenderloin 300g	Pink Himalayan rock salt
Salmon steak x 180g	Epsom salts x 1 packet
Protein powder of your choice	Avocado x 2
Almonds x 1 packet	Baby spinach x 1 packet
Eggs large – 1 dozen	Frozen mixed berries
Greek Yoghurt 1kg tub	Bananas x small bunch
Extra lean beef mince x 500g	Dijon mustard
White fish x 180g	Macadamia oil 1 bottle
Red capsicum x 2 large	Lettuce – any type or mixed leaf
Yellow capsicum x 2 large	Cherry tomatoes x 2 punnets
Green capsicum x 2 large	Lemons x 6 large
Broccolini x 1 bunch	Ginger x 1 root
Roma tomatoes x 5	Apple Cider Vinegar x 1 bottle
Asparagus x 1 bunch	Cinnamon x 1 packet of
Spanish onions x 4	Cayenne pepper x 1 packet
Mushrooms	Zucchini
Green beans x 200g	Carrots x 1 bag
Celery x half bunch	Oats x 1 packet

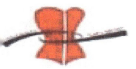

To make food preparation easier - choose 3 or 4 main meals that you enjoy eating. Multiply the ingredients and adjust your shopping list accordingly. Allocate one day a week to food preparation. Prepare your meals in bulk and portion in to containers for each meal. You will be less likely to succumb to cravings when you have your healthy meals on hand. A bonus will be the time you save each evening not having to cook daily.

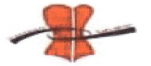

Chapter 4: Turn your body into a fat melting machine

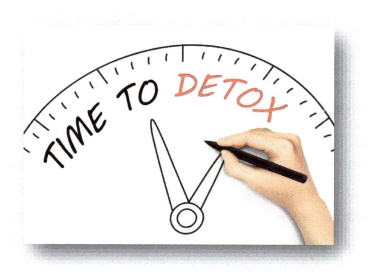

Phase 1: Carb Detox

Fair warning: the first couple of days are going to bring some unpleasant reactions. Changing your lifestyle and way of eating is not easy. So, we are going to do this in steps. It is important that you transition from your old habits into this new clean way of health and nutrition carefully. To do this, we must first cleanse our body out of toxins and inflammation. Our bodies have stored and trapped toxins inside our fat cells.

Once we stop feeding our bodies the wrong types of foods, these trapped toxins will be released out of the body through every pore and lymph node. The main culprit here is going to be the addiction to sugar. With addictiveness like cocaine, quitting sugar can come with it a host of not-so-fun withdrawal symptoms. These may appear in different intensity levels for different people. Stay with it – take paracetamol and see your doctor but stick with it – it's well worth the effort to get to the other side.

Yes, sucrose is one addictive beast and it won't let go of you without a fight. Plus, the temptation will be everywhere, so stay strong. The best is yet to come but not before the headaches. Much like when you give up that other addictive vice, caffeine, headaches are a very commonly reported symptom of sugar withdrawal. Time to invest in some aromatherapy oils, and make sure to drink plenty of water. At this point, your brain receptors are going to be screaming: Chocolate, cakes biscuits anything with SUGAR! Between that, the headaches and the cravings, you may understandably have some pretty severe mood swings. It's helpful to have a solid support network around you during this stage, to help you remember why you started.

But suddenly, you'll come out the other side feeling better than ever. It could be a few days or a week, it varies person to person; however, once you do get through this bumpy stage, your body will no longer crave sugar. You will not experience the sugar highs and 3pm crashes – which is how sugar behaves in your body. Instead, you will have a steady energy level, less mood swings, clearer skin and start to notice a drop in your weight. Usually, the first week you will drop weight quickly just by clearing the inflammation.

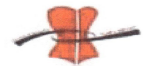

Ok? Are you ready to start?

Remember you are not alone on this.

Join our community on our Facebook page:

https://www.facebook.com/ketowithsarahjane

To begin the 3-day detox, please follow the directions below:

Each morning when you awake and before your breakfast, drink a glass of warm water and a tablespoon of apple cider vinegar. The warm water will start your metabolism working after your restorative sleep. The apple cider vinegar has multiple researched benefits such as balancing your ph. in the body and a natural fat burner.

You may also like to compound your results with the "morning kick start' in the recipe section

For the next 3 days we are going to supercharge your results by doing an elimination detox. This elimination detox requires you to literally strip back all the foods in your diet that may have caused you your symptoms. Only then will we have a clean slate.

You will eat a protein-only diet for 3 days*. Drink plenty of lemon water and take a good vitamin/mineral supplement. *Please note that this is only TEMPORARY to serve an important function.

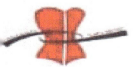

The reason we are doing protein only is that fruits are simple carbohydrates containing fructose (or sugar) and many vegetables also contain levels of carbohydrates. We are aiming to maximize the detoxification and wean ourselves off carbohydrates. This method is the best way to do this. The other method is fasting. This will allow our body to deplete glucose levels in it and trigger ketosis which I will explain in later chapters. After these 3 days, we are then going to introduce back into our diet the right types of macro nutrients and nutrition to feed and nourish your body. What you will find is once you get through this you will absolutely love to eat vegetables/salads even if you never had before!

It is very important that you plan and pre-prepare your protein meals for the next 3 days. You WILL have cravings and you will need to have protein on hand to eat when they do hit. Preparation is the absolute key to success. Cook ahead and portion your meals out. This will ensure you won't ruin your efforts.

For your main meals and snacks, you are going to choose any source of lean protein. See the list on the next page. Do not use protein shakes or protein bars at this stage – They contain hidden sugars.

No starches (Complex carbohydrates) – That is NO rice, pasta, potatoes, chips, or bread.

No sugars (Simple carbohydrates) – no fruit, (some vegetables. E.g. sweet potatoes, peas, and carrots are grouped as starchy vegetables so watch your intake of those).

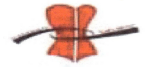

Protein

Good choices of protein are:

- Seafood.
- Chicken breast
- Turkey
- White Fish
- Salmon
- Milk
- Cottage cheese
- Greek Yogurt.
- Egg whites.
- Beans
- Pork Tenderloin
- Lean Beef.

For these 3 days, you must maintain a– **Low carbohydrate diet**. and keep **sugars as close to ZERO** as you can.

Stay away from packaged meals - they have hidden sugars and all sorts of chemicals added that you are aiming to wean yourself from.

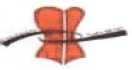

With the protein, portion sizes vary with men and women and body size. For most people, a daily dose of around 0.8-1g of protein per 1kg of body weight is recommended. However, for simplicity, the general rule of thumb is the size of your palm

The method of cooking your protein is also important so the preferred options are baking, grilling, steaming, etc.

Water

Also, watch what you drink – Water only – no soft drinks, no fruit juice, no flavored milks, energy drinks, etc. If you used to drink coffees or tea, be mindful of adding milk and sugar - use artificial sugar or better still, go without.

To detox the body, we need to assist the body in that process by helping it to flush through the kidneys and digestive system and out. Therefore, you are going to have to drink plenty of water.

So, if you have a gallon container – fill that up at the start of each day – this is a visual technique to remind you that you must drink all of it. If not, then 2 x 2 Litre containers.

The 2nd day reduces to 3 Litres and the 3rd day back to 2 Litres.

This is a large volume of water than most of you would drink. It is only for these 3 days of the detox. You will find that you frequently visit the bathroom.

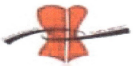

Sauna session

To step up the detoxification process, you can do a sauna session. A sauna stimulates the removal of toxins from the body and improves the circulation and cleanses the whole body. Saunas also assist in weight loss.

When you use a sauna, follow the following basic safety rules:

- Keep your session to a maximum of 30 minutes at a time.
- Ensure you drink plenty of water before and after the session.
- Rest lying or sitting for approximately 10 minutes afterwards.
- Do not use a sauna if you are pregnant, have hypertension, hyperthyroidism or any kind of heart condition.
- When you have finished in the sauna take a shower.

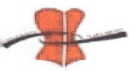

Epsom salt bath

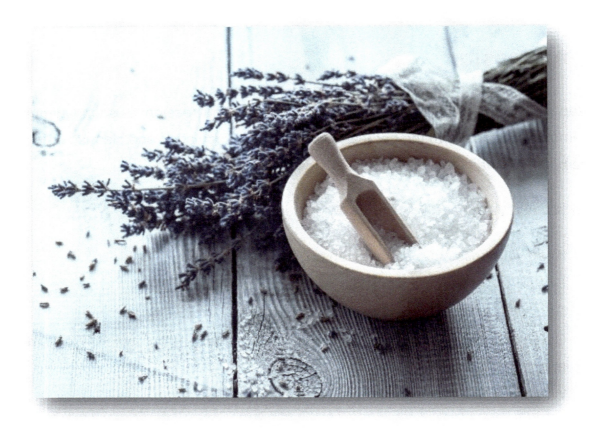

If you do not have access to a sauna, you can get similar effect just taking a warm bath and adding Epsom salts. Epsom salts are available from most pharmacies or selected supermarkets. Epsom salts are a naturally occurring mineral compound of magnesium and sulfate. It is known as a natural remedy for several ailments and it has numerous health benefits, many studies have shown that magnesium and sulfate are both readily absorbed through the skin, making a bath with Epsom salts an easy and effective way to enjoy the benefits such as:

- ✓ Eliminates toxins from the body
- ✓ Eases stress
- ✓ Improves sleep
- ✓ Relieves constipation
- ✓ Improves absorption of nutrients
- ✓ Relieves pain and muscle cramps
- ✓ Prevents and eases migraine headaches
- ✓ Regulates electrolytes
- ✓ Relaxes the nervous system
- ✓ Treats colds and congestion

Fill the bath with warm water that is hot to the touch but not burning. Add 1 – 2 cups of Epsom salts to your bath depending on your size/weight. As with the sauna sessions – ensure you check with your physician and follow basic safety pre-cautions. Drink plenty of water before and after.

Make sure you monitor your progress. Stand on the scales on Day 1 of the detox and record your results on the final day 3. Most people will see a shift on the scales. Some will say it's just water weight. True to an extent that toxins and carbohydrates hold onto water in the body. So, detoxing will help this move out of the body.

Also look at yourself in the mirror – does your stomach appear less bloated, etc. Not everything is about numbers – sometimes, it's how you feel, maybe your skin looks better, eyes are brighter, moods have improved, energy increased, etc.

Once you have successfully gotten through the carb detox period, you will now re-introduce fruits and vegetables back into your diet as well as healthy fats. This will be further explained as we work towards implementing a ketogenic diet to burn fats including body fat as fuel.

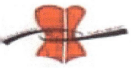

Natural Fat Burners

Elevate your fat burning to the next level by incorporating any of these natural fats burning ingredients into your regular diet and nutritional plan.

Ginger

Ginger is a root known for its numerous health properties. Its anti-inflammatory properties help the digestive system. Ginger also expands the blood vessels allowing more blood to flow. This increases the heat supplied around the fat tissues by 20% hence burning it off. Ginger can be added in tea or mixed with lime juice.

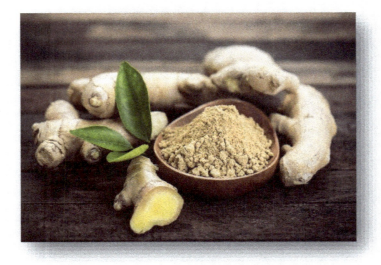

Cayenne Pepper

Cayenne pepper has a chemical compound called capsaicin. It is known to reduce the amount of fat stored in the body by altering the absorption rate of fat cells. Cayenne pepper also contains high levels of Vitamin C which accelerate the metabolism of the body allowing it to burn fat more quickly.

Green Tea

Although the caffeine content in Green Tea contributes to making it a reliable fat burner, what really makes it effective is the presence of Catechins and antioxidants. They have a fat-reducing effect which has been proven by multiple studies. It works by reducing the body's ability to absorb fats from foods by 35% to 43%.

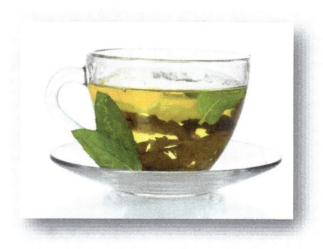

Nuts

Nuts such as almonds are known to work well when mixed with other foods such as yoghurt and oatmeal. A study published in the *International Journal of Obesity* showed that participants who had almonds daily for at least six months lost about 18% of their body fat.

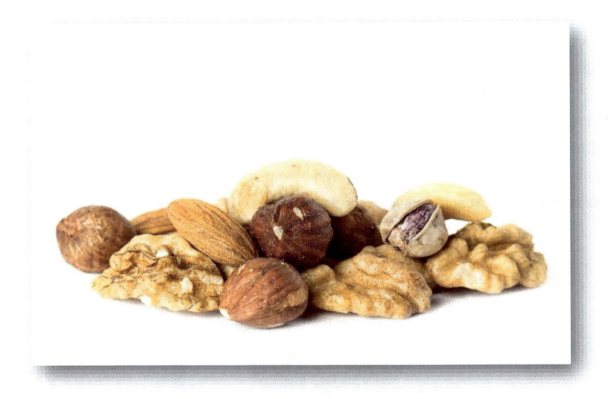

Berries

Berries such as; blueberries, strawberries and raspberries contain a compound known as polyphenol. This compound is a powerful natural chemical that burns excess fat in the body. Studies performed on mice at Texas Women's University showed that this compound reduced the formation of fat cells by up to 73%.

Grapefruit

Rich in antioxidants, vitamins, lycopene and fibre, grapefruit also detoxifies and can help you lose weight. Grapefruit, with its bitter sweetness, is a popular citrus fruit commonly eaten for breakfast to help kick-start digestion and aid in weight loss. This refreshing fruit could also hold the key to treating conditions such as high cholesterol and type 2 diabetes. Researchers from the Hebrew University of Jerusalem and Massachusetts General Hospital have recently found that naringenin, an antioxidant derived from bitter-flavoured grapefruit and other citrus fruits, may cause the liver to break down fat while increasing insulin sensitivity, mimicking the actions of lipid-lowering and anti-diabetic drugs. Naringenin may also protect against liver damage.

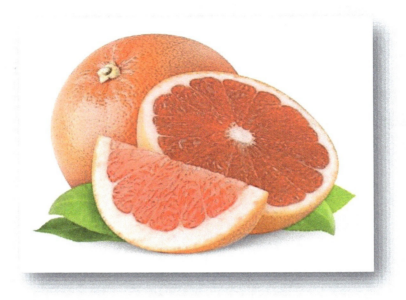

Greek Yoghurt

Greek yoghurt has a high content of calcium which is known to inhibit the production of cortisol – a hormone that promotes accumulation of fat in the abdomen. Greek yoghurt is classified as low-fat dairy products which can help people reduce weight.

Apple Cider Vinegar

Acetic acid, one of the major components of apple cider vinegar, may help with weight loss because it may suppress fat accumulation. Consuming a daily dose of vinegar led to a lower body weight, waist circumference and abdominal fat mass, according to a 2009 study published in Bioscience, Biotechnology and Biochemistry. Researchers hypothesized that the acetic acid was responsible for the change.

Green Vegetables (Kale, Spinach and Broccoli)

Cruciferous vegetables like cauliflower, spinach, kale and broccoli are nutritionally dense vegetables. They are high in Vitamin A and potassium. Potassium can help LOWER insulin resistance (Awesome news) These vegetables are full of '*Phytonutrients*' these are the trace minerals that can fight cancer.

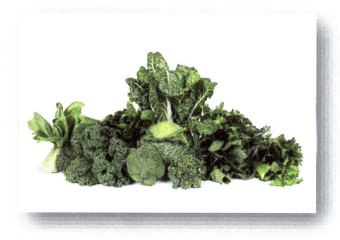

Cinnamon

Cinnamon is very effective in burning fat; especially visceral fat – which is stored in the belly area. It contains a compound called cinnamaldehyde which gives it its flavor. This compound stimulates metabolism of the fatty visceral tissue hence reducing fat. It is also known to control blood sugar by maintaining insulin sensitivity.

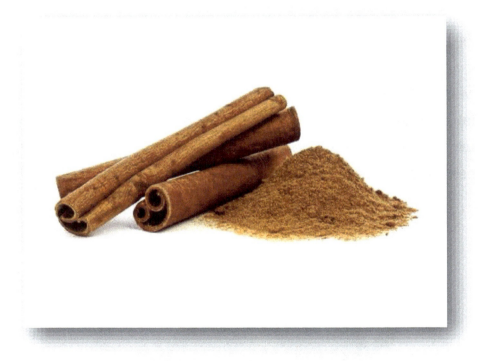

Avocado

Avocadoes are rich in mono-unsaturated and oleic fatty acids which have been proven to reduce fat in the belly area. A diet rich in mono-saturated fats prevents body fat distribution around the belly. Avocado oil-regulates the expression of some fat genes.

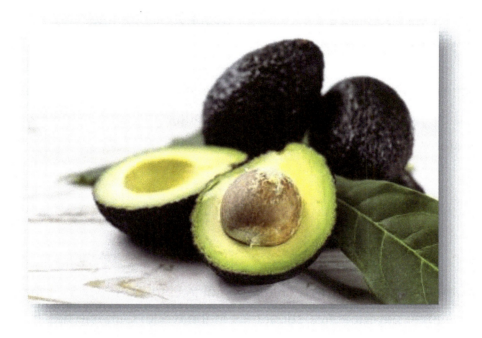

Chiai Seeds

As a nutritional powerhouse, Chiai seeds are also considered as one of the most effective fat-burning foods. This food, originally grown in Mexico, contains so much water which helps slow down the body's digestion hence reducing hunger pangs and sugar cravings. They also provide the body with high energy and more endurance power.

Coconut Oil

Coconut oil has long been known as a source of medium chain saturated fatty acids which are very effective in fighting weight gain. It boosts metabolism and provides a lot of energy that helps in burning extra calories. Coconut oil promotes the natural detoxification of the body by metabolizing fats in the liver.

It can be taken right after dinner or in place of olive oil. A tablespoon twice a day is recommended by most nutritionists. You can also add a tablespoon to herbal tea, lemon juice or hot water.

Coffee

We all love our coffee and know that coffee contains caffeine… which is the most commonly consumed psychoactive substance in the world. Caffeine has made its way to most commercial fat burning supplements, for a good reason. It is one of the few substances that are known to help mobilize fats from the fat tissues and increase metabolism. In fact, coffee contains several biologically active substances that can affect metabolism:

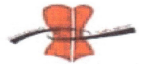

- ➢ Caffeine– a central nervous system stimulant.
- ➢ Theobromine and Theophylline– substances related to caffeine that can also have a stimulant effect.
- ➢ Chlorogenic Acid– one of the biologically active compounds in coffee, may help slow absorption of carbohydrates.

Coffee, just like green tea, has fat-burning qualities that translate into big losses in calories over time. It increases the Basal Metabolic Rate (discussed in earlier chapters) In fact, the caffeine in just one cup can boost calorie burning by four percent over the course of two and half hours.

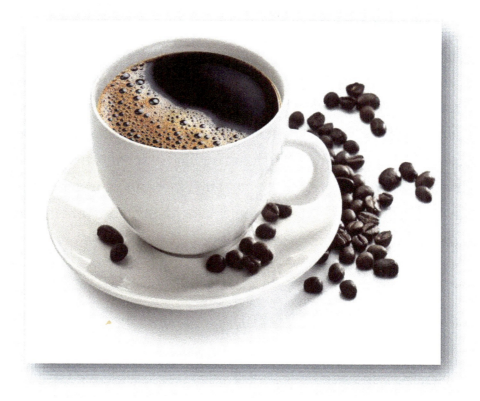

Garcinia Cambrogia

Garcinia Cambrogia has been clinically proven to help with weight loss as well as cleanse the body. Detox is an essential part of weight loss. It is often the first step which helps clear your body and its pathways, such as colons, of toxins. Garcinia Cambrogia is a natural cleanser which also has other proven health benefits such as; relieving stomach discomforts, reducing appetite and blocking accumulation of fat.

Beta Hydroxy-butyrate (Exogenous Ketone supplement)

Beta Hydroxy-butyrate or BHB is an essential component of the ketone bodies. It promotes ketosis in the body which boosts weight loss. Essentially, it works by unlocking the fat cells and converting it into an energy source instead of glucose (Carbohydrates). We'll discuss this in detail in Chapter 7 of this book. It comes in the form of a supplement and is a very effective fat burning mechanism since it is very hard to find the right combination of foods or the right diet that can jumpstart ketosis in the body. It is ideal for practically all sorts of people. Whether you are a body builder, a regular dieter or someone with abnormal fat cells.

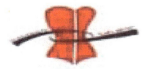

I'm Sick of Being Fat! – Sarah Jane

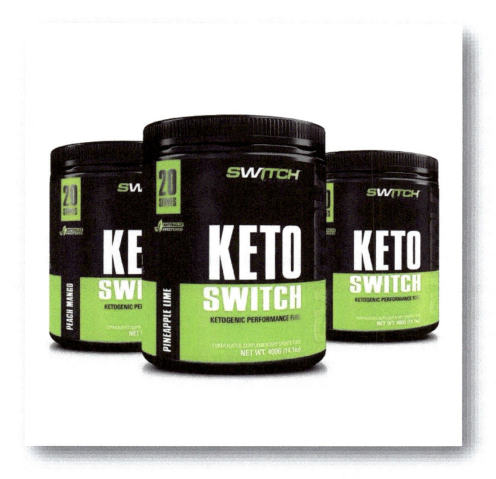

Green Supplements

Green supplements are helpful if you don't consume enough raw vegetables in your diet. Your body needs various vitamins and minerals. Your body will disfunction if it is depleted of these essential vitamins and minerals. So, if you don't generally eat enough vegetables a green supplement may be what you need.

Metabolism Boosting Recipes

Miracle Weight Loss Tea

This miracle weight loss tea utilizes several of the best fat burners to melt off that fat. This tea is recommended to have after your evening meal and before bed time. Some of the known benefits include;

- ACV contains acetic acid which Improves metabolic rate of the body.
- Boosts energy levels to help with weight loss.
- Contains a lot of anti-oxidants which help cleanse the body.
- Cinnamon helps regulate blood sugar levels to stop those spikes.

Ingredients:

- Grated lemon zest and juice of 1 lemon
- Ginger from the root – grated or finely chopped
- ¼ Teaspoon cayenne pepper
- ½ Teaspoon cinnamon
- 1 Tablespoon apple cider vinegar
- Hot water

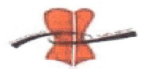

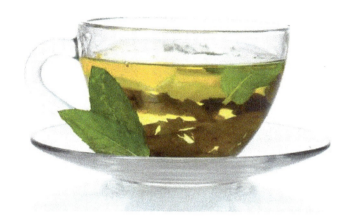

Morning 'Metabolism kick starter'

Every day on-rising, before your breakfast, drink the following;

- 1 glass of WARM water with:
- 2 Tablespoons of Apple cider vinegar
- Juice of 1 lemon
- ½ teaspoon of cinnamon

The ACV helps to de-alkalize your body, lemon and warm water helps to detoxify and get your digestive system working efficiently, the cinnamon will help to regulate your blood sugar levels throughout the day to prevent those spikes from happening and assists in the taste. – Yes, it is an acquired taste – but stick with it – the results far outweigh the taste.

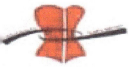

'Keto Mocha Coffee'/a.k.a – 'Bullet proof' coffee

- 1 scoop of coffee – either French pressed or espresso
- Hot water
- 1 Tablespoon of MCT oil or coconut oil
- ½ teaspoon of cinnamon
- 1/2 scoop of Keto-Switch chocolate ketones

Method:

Place in a heat proof high speed blender and blend for a few seconds until combined.

The fat burning properties of coffee are increased when blended with the MCT fats to get into your cells fast. The cinnamon replicates insulin in the body and therefore balances out your blood sugar levels. This will mean fewer cravings for sugar and no energy pikes and troughs.

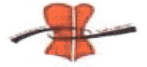

Green Smoothie

Healthy smoothies improve digestion and can help with weight loss. Green Tea Smoothie is ideal for those who like green tea. It is made by mixing the following ingredients:

- ¾-cup chilled green tea
- 1 teaspoon of green supplement
- 1 banana
- ¼-cup non-fat plain Greek yoghurt
- 1 Tablespoon of MCT oil or coconut oil
- Couple of drops of stevia
- ½-cup baby spinach
- This smoothie is a weight loss miracle because it combines all essential foods that help with weight loss.

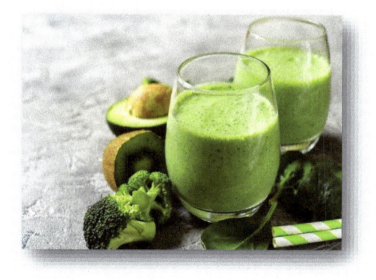

Triple Berry Blast

The Triple Berry Blast is a delicious smoothie; it consists of the following ingredients;

- 1 cup frozen and unsweetened blueberries
- 1 cup frozen and unsweetened raspberries
- 1 cup halved strawberries
- 1 scoop of vanilla protein powder
- 1 cup unsweetened Almond Milk
- 4-5 ice cubes

All the ingredients are mixed and blended together until smooth.

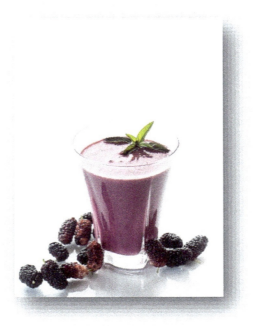

Keto Chocolate Mousse

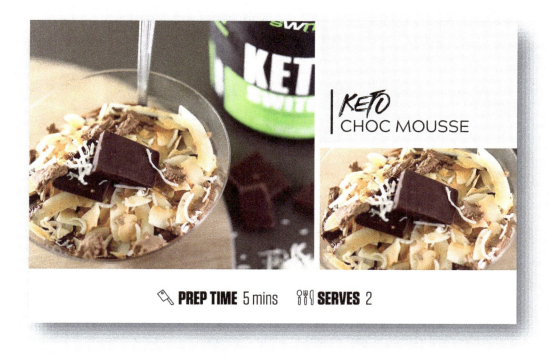

Ingredients

- 1 large Avocado
- 2 tbsp. Cacao Powder
- 1 scoop Keto Switch - Chocolate
- 1/2 cup Coconut Cream
- 50g melted Dark Chocolate
- 1/2 tsp. Vanilla Extract

Method

1. Mix all ingredients in a blender until smooth.
2. Serve topped with fresh Fruit, Chocolate Chunks, Shredded Coconut, etc.

The bonus, aside from being delicious – also ==kicks you into ketosis in 30 mins.==

Quick Fat-Burner Salad

There is a great deal of fat-burner salad recipes to choose from and many of which are quite healthy and delicious. The Super Raw Power Salad, for example, brings together all foods low in carbs and rich in nutrients and minerals.

Ingredients:

- 4 cups of finely chopped kale
- 1½ cups chopped purple cabbage
- ¾-cup dried berries and/or tart cherries
- ½-cup raw sunflower seeds
- ½-cup mung bean
- 2 chopped apples
- Salt and pepper to taste

The dressing is made of the following ingredients'

- ¾-cup Macadamia nut oil (if allergies subst. extra virgin olive oil
- ¼-cup apple cider vinegar
- 1 teaspoon Dijon mustard
- ¼ teaspoon garlic powder
- salt and pepper to taste

Café Mocha Smoothie

This milkshake tastes like you're eating ice cream but with all the health benefits. Full of protein and satiating fibre plus the extra kick of fat burning ketosis

- ¾ cup chilled brewed coffee
- 1 banana
- ½ cup almond milk
- 1 scoop vanilla or chocolate protein powder
- ½ scoop of chocolate flavoured 'Keto-switch'

Method:

In a blender, combine all ingredients with ½ cup of ice. Blend until frothy, about 1 minute.

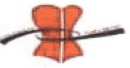

Breakfast Bowl

It is important to jumpstart your day with a meal loaded with vitamins, antioxidants, fibers and minerals. Take for instance the Super Food Chocolate Breakfast Bowl recipe.

Ingredients:

- 1 scoop of chocolate protein
- ½-cup unsweetened Almond milk
- 2 tablespoons of Greek yoghurt
- 1 teaspoon Cacao powder
- ½-cup frozen blueberries
- ½-cup banana

  Topping options include;

- 2 tablespoons quinoa crisps
- 1 tablespoon Chiai seeds
- 1 tablespoon slivered almonds or coconut flakes
- ½-banana sliced

Blend the base ingredients together until smooth. Pour into a bowl then add the toppings however you see fit and enjoy your breakfast bowl.

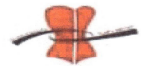

Protein Pancakes

Copyright: recipe: Sarah Jane

Ingredients:

- 2 scoops of good quality vanilla protein powder (use whey -avoid soy protein isolate)
- 1 egg white
- 1 tablespoon of MCT oil (or coconut oil)
- 1 tsp. cinnamon
- 1 teaspoon of liquid 'stevia'
- 1/3 cup of water

*For extra kick and additional taste – why not add ½ scoop of raspberry/peach or chocolate flavoured ketone supplement like <u>Keto switch</u>

Method:

1. Mix protein powder, egg white, and MCT oil together, add water gradually to smooth out lumps and to create a thick batter-like consistency.
2. Cook on a medium heat in a non-stick fry pan; use a small spoonful of coconut oil for cooking. Add your favorite natural toppings like healthy blueberries, strawberries and mangos.

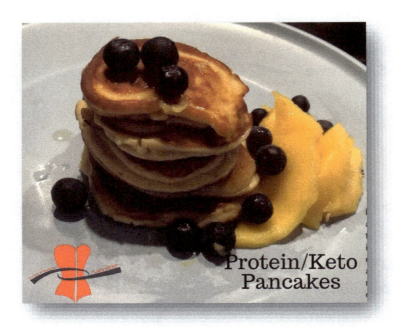

Keto -Friendly Mayonnaise

Copyright: Recipe: Sarah Jane

Ingredients:

- 1 egg
- 1 heaped Tsp. Dijon mustard
- 1 Tsp. minced garlic
- Pinch of pink Himalayan Salt
- 1 small pinch cayenne pepper (good for fat burning)
- 1 Tablespoon of Apple Cider Vinegar
- 350ml of MCT oil

Method:

In a bowl, mix the egg, mustard, garlic S&P, and gradually add the MCT oil until it thickens. Season to taste, add more vinegar if required, or add more oil to thicken.

(MCT oil can also be substituted for Macadamia Oil)

This recipe is my go-to for all my salads. It allows me to keep up my good fats for my macros and has the added health benefits without any of the manufactured additives, colours, etc.

Use the same recipe base without the egg for a standard French style dressing.

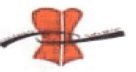

Keto Panna Cotta

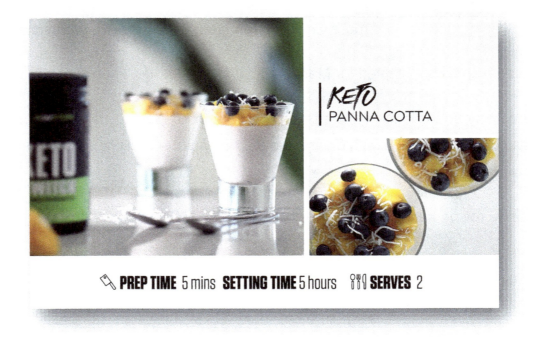

Ingredients

- 1 can Coconut Cream
- 1 tbsp. Grass-fed Gelatin
- 1 serve Keto Switch Peach Mango
- 1/2 tsp. Vanilla Extract
- Fresh Mango
- Shredded Coconut

Method

1. Whisk Gelatin with 1/2 cup Coconut Cream and let sit for 5 minutes.
2. Heat over low heat until the Gelatin dissolves (do not boil).
3. Add the remaining ingredients and stir.
4. Pour into glasses or ramekins.
5. Set for 5 hours in the fridge or overnight.
6. Top with fresh Mango and Shredded Coconut to serve.

Keto 'Berry' delicious Mousse

Copyright: Recipe: Sarah Jane

Ingredients

- 1 packet of gelatin leaves approx. 7 small or 3 large.
- 500 ml of boiling water
- 500ml cold water
- 6 scoops of Raspberry flavored 'Keto-Switch'
- 1 punnet of assorted berries – use fresh or frozen blueberries, strawberries raspberries
- 2 x 500g cottage cheese

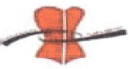

Method

1. First boil the water, measure out (500ml) and add to the gelatin. Mix until all the gelatin has dissolved.
2. Measure out 500 ml of cold water and add your keto switch until dissolved.
3. Add your keto-switch and water to the fruit. Using a blender or food processor to blend all the fruit with the water to create a smooth coulis /fruit puree.
4. Add the dissolved gelatin to the berry coulis and mix well.
5. Place the cottage cheese into a large bowl and slowly add the berry coulis. Mix well until you get a smooth consistency using a stick mixer (You can also do this in a blender if capacity allows).
6. Pour the mix into small containers and refrigerate for 5 hours or overnight. Enjoy!

Believe me, it is berry delicious! You could also blend up some almonds or macadamias, mix with coconut oil and set it as a base then add your mousse for a Keto Berry cheesecake!

High in antioxidants, high in protein, low sugar and puts you into fat burning state of ketosis in 30 mins!

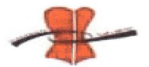

Keto Coconut Pineapple & lime "Weis Bars"

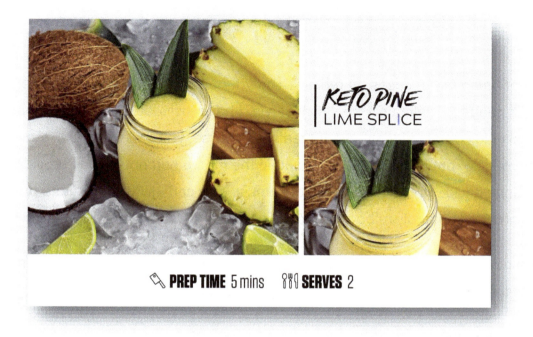

- 2 cups chopped fresh Pineapple
- 1 cup Coconut Milk
- 1 serve Keto Switch - Pineapple Lime
- Juice of half a fresh Lime
- **Ice**

Method

1. Blend all ingredients until smooth and top with mint. NOTE: Add more water as needed.
2. Set in ice block molds for a refreshing icy treat!

Chapter 5: Daily Meal Plans

"I'm sick of being fat!" focuses on replenishing your body with the vital and essential nutrients it needs to maintain a healthy lifestyle. I have included a 7-day plan that you can use to guide you in planning your meals. Of course, you can tweak this template however you like, but remember to stay within the macro nutrient ranges provided so that you don't accidently get kicked out of ketosis. You can always substitute protein sources, greens, metabolism boosting foods and natural fat burners.

The main goal is to change your eating from processed foods to sources that are true to its natural form as possible. This is often referred to as 'Clean eating'.

Your meals are going to be structured during the day as:

1. Breakfast,
2. Lunch
3. Dinner

As you progress with this programme we will eventually move you towards Intermittent fasting which will supercharge your fat loss results. So, try to ensure you DON'T snack as this spikes insulin.

Quantities on the following meal plans have not been listed as they vary with men and women, body weight as well as level of activity. For most people, a daily dose of around 0.8-1g of protein per 1kg of body weight is recommended.

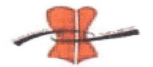

As we progress further into a keto diet you will eventually decrease the number of meals eaten per day down to one or 2 with the intermittent fasting, but for now we are just taking small steps at a time towards gaining health.

Also aim to go for a 30-minute brisk walk before your first meal of the day. It activates your body's fat burning mechanism by accelerating the fat burning process of the stored fat. Take your exogenous ketone supplement on an empty stomach before you start your morning exercise. This is often referred to as 'Fasted Cardio' and will speed up your results.

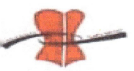

7-Day Meal Plan

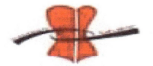

Day 1

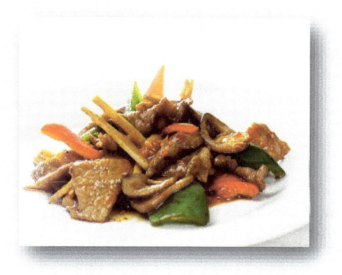

On rising: 200ml of warm water with apple cider vinegar

1 x *Keto-switch'* with 200ml water

Breakfast
3 x eggs tomatoes, mushrooms, Spanish onion, baby spinach leaves

Lunch
Beef stir fry: sautéed lean beef strip steamed snow peas, red and yellow capsicum, green beans, carrots and a handful of raw nuts (cashews, almonds macadamias or walnuts)

Afternoon
1 x 'Keto-switch' with 200ml water
Dinner

Chicken breast grilled with lemon and herbs Cherry tomatoes, Broccolini

DAY 2

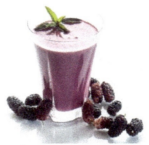

On rising: 200ml of warm water with apple cider vinegar

1 x 'Keto-switch' with 200ml water
Breakfast

Smoothie made with chocolate or vanilla protein powder
1/4 cup mixed berries
1 spoonful of LSA
1/4 teaspoon of cinnamon
150ml of water or almond milk, ice cubes

Lunch

2 x Beef rissoles - made from lean beef mince with Italian herbs, garlic, egg, salt and pepper
1/4 Avocado, tomato, Spanish(red) onion, roasted pumpkin or sweet potato

Dinner
Lean cut of rump steak
Broccoli, sweet potato, zucchini

Day 3

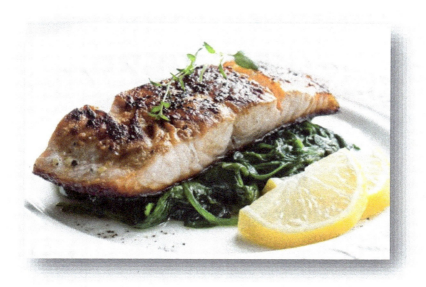

On rising: 200ml of warm water with apple cider vinegar

'1 x 'Keto-switch' with 200ml water

Breakfast
Frittata - 3 x eggs
Chopped capsicums, shallots, tomato, mushrooms

Lunch
Canned tuna
Salad with lettuce, 1/4 Avocado, cucumber, Spanish (red) onion, tomato, capsicum, with balsamic vinaigrette.
1 x 'Keto-switch' with 200ml water
Dinner
Salmon steak grilled with herbs, lemon and S&P Steamed asparagus, sweet potato

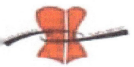

Day 4

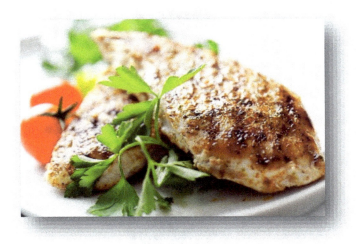

On rising; 200ml of warm water with apple cider vinegar

1 x 'Keto-switch' with 200ml water

Breakfast

3x eggs
tomato, mushrooms, Spanish onion, baby spinach leaves

Snack

Lunch

Canned tuna mixed salad with avocado, tomato, Spanish onion, capsicum and balsamic vinaigrette

Snack

1 x 'Keto-switch' with 200ml water

Dinner

Chicken breast sprinkled with paprika, turmeric, S&P steamed green beans, broccoli, zucchini, roasted sweet potato

Day 5

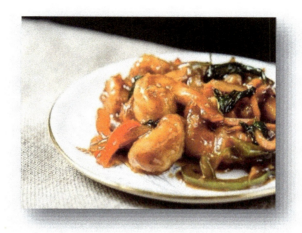

On rising: 200ml of warm water with apple cider vinegar

1 x 'Keto-switch' with 200ml water
Breakfast
   Smoothie made with: 1 scoop of chocolate flavoured protein

- 1 scoop of chocolate Keto-switch'
- 150ml of coconut water or almond milk with a handful of ice cubes

Lunch

Grilled chicken salad with baby spinach leaves, avocado, tomato, cucumber Spanish onion, vinaigrette dressing.

Snack
1 x 'Keto-switch' with 200ml water

Dinner
Prawns sautéed with garlic and green beans, cashew nuts, Spanish onions, sliced capsicums.

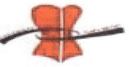

Day 6

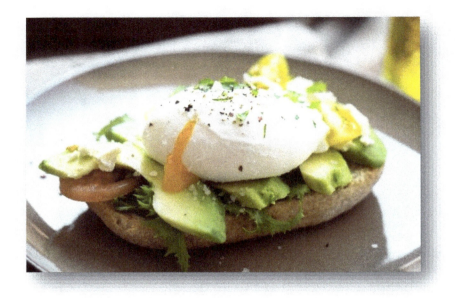

On rising: 200ml of warm water with freshly squeezed lemon

1 x 'Keto-switch' with 200ml water

Breakfast

3 x poached eggs with seasoned avocado, baby spinach leaves and tomatoes

Lunch

lean beef burger patties with salad of lettuce, cucumber, cherry tomatoes, avocado and capsicum - balsamic vinaigrette

Snack

handful of macadamia nuts

1 x 'Keto-switch' with 200ml water

Dinner

Salmon steak lightly pan fried with lemon and cracked pepper, sea salt blanched fresh asparagus and sweet potato

Day 7

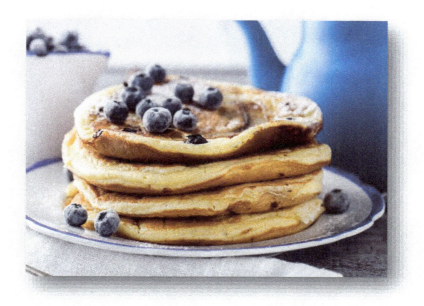

On rising: 200ml of warm water with apple cider vinegar

1 x 'Keto-switch' with 200ml water

Breakfast
Protein pancakes (See recipe add toppings such as fresh blueberries, strawberries and a sprinkle of cinnamon)

Lunch
Warm garlic beef strip salad tossed with snow peas, cherry tomatoes, cucumbers, baby spinach and rocket leaves drizzled with extra virgin olive oil.

Snack
1 x 'Keto-switch' with 200ml water

Dinner
White fish fillet lightly pan-fried with lemon and S&P Steamed snow peas, cherry tomatoes, avocado

Chapter 6: Ketosis and the Ketogenic diet

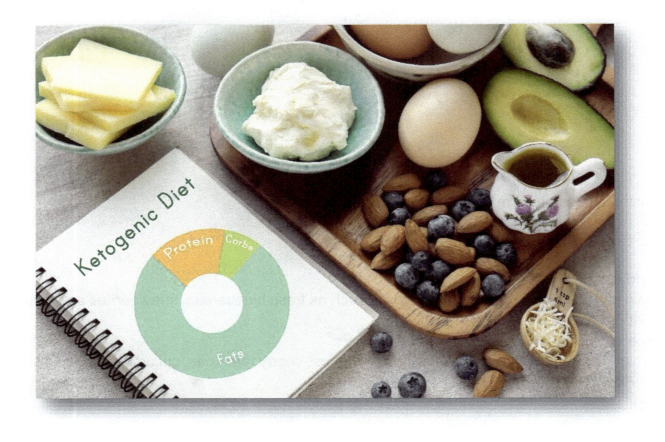

What is Ketosis?

In order to help you understand more, the ketogenic diet and what is involved, you may like to watch my introductory video using the link below. This will help you prepare for what's ahead.

https://www.youtube.com/watch?v=OccowDdcSpk&t=19s

The ketogenic diet is not new and has been in practice since 1920. It involves following a low carbohydrate (10%), moderate protein (20%) and high fat (70%) diet. (A.K.A - LCHF). The ketogenic diet first became popular as a treatment for seizures in children suffering from epilepsy, and the neuro-protective benefits of ketones came to light. As research into the process of ketosis now expands, the list of benefits just continues to grow.

When it comes to adopting a ketogenic diet, focus is usually on consuming less carbs and allowing the body to burn the stored fat in your body as energy. However, a proper ketogenic diet takes so much more into account than just the carbs. It also involves avoiding processed foods that could contain harmful toxins.

The human body is intriguing in many ways, especially when it comes to the production of energy for everyday normal functions.

This energy can come from two (2) sources:

1. the burning of glucose /carbohydrates
2. Or the burning of fat. (including stored body fat)

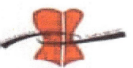

This is what many refer to as ketosis, a state where the body obtains its fuel from burning the fat stored in it. The body will often resort to burning fat when there is little to no glucose in it, making it a last resort when creating energy for the entire body or a native source of fuel.

Ideally, if the levels of glucose or the amount of carbs are low enough in the body, it will automatically switch to the breaking down of the fat stored in the body as a source of energy. This is where the benefits of ketosis truly shine through, especially regarding weight loss. When the body is forced to turn to the stored fat to create energy, excess fat that contributed to weight gain is lost in the process. Ketosis therefore becomes an interesting way to cut down on unnecessary fat in the body, making it a popular weight loss strategy for many people.

On top of cutting down on the body weight, ketosis also results in reduced cravings for food, thanks to a curbed appetite. With a suppressed appetite, it is easy to avoid the unnecessary eating and snacking that is often the cause of excess weight gain. There are so many more benefits that come with ketosis which will come further in this book, but on top of the main benefits that are weight loss and improved body composition, the rest are welcome bonuses.

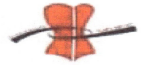

The Basics of a Ketogenic Diet

Reducing carbohydrate intake

The main purpose of a ketogenic diet is to help your body get used to processing fats for energy. Carbohydrates in the form of starchy carbs/grains are therefore to be avoided at all costs. Most grains such as wheat, rye, quinoa, bread, rice, cakes, cookies, crackers, biscuits and various others are to be avoided. Sugars and sweets are notorious for their high calorie contents and should also be put away. It is also worth noting that most high calorie foods come from processed food, and should also be avoided at all costs

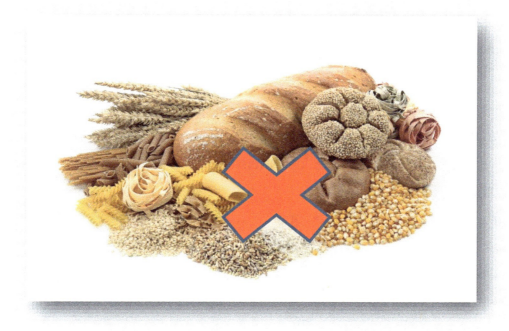

Increasing 'Good Fat' Intake

At a glance, this may sound counterintuitive since you are trying to lose weight by burning fat in the first place. However, a healthy ketogenic diet should also help your body adapt to breaking down fats to produce energy. Since the principal source of energy for your body is fat, it is important to focus on eating foods rich in fat. The kind of fat also matters, as unhealthy fats are counterproductive towards the weight loss goal. Some of the ideal recommended foods include avocados for the mono-saturated fat and omega 3 from seafood and the saturated fats that come from butter and coconut oil.

Balancing out salt or sodium intake

When the body is more focused on carbs as a source of energy, a lot of sodium is often released into the body. When the diet shifts to one focusing more on fats instead, the salt content in the body reduces drastically. It is therefore important to incorporate foods that add a bit of sodium to the system to balance out the expected deficiency. These include carrots, celery and meat. Also ensure that you always use Pink Himalayan salt. This salt has been found to contain up to 80 different essential minerals that your body need. So contrary to beliefs about salt, this type of salt – not the processed table salt variety is good for your body.

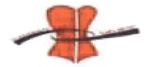

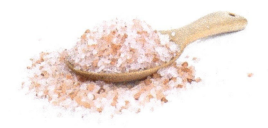

Don't forget the vegetables

Most diets that contribute to weight loss often have the added benefit of also improving the overall body health. This principle also rings true for a ketogenic diet. Non-starchy vegetables like spinach, lettuce, chives, asparagus and cucumbers come highly recommended for their vitamin value.

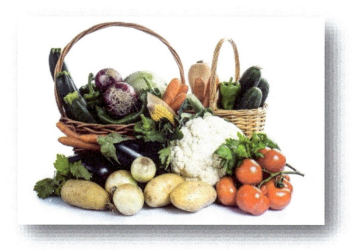

Timing

A ketogenic can often be utilized with 'intermittent fasting' for far more effective results. All the meals that are to be consumed for the day for an individual following a ketogenic diet should be done so within a 6-hour window. This prevents overeating and allows the body more time to focus on burning body fat for energy. It is important that all eating be done a minimum of 3 hours before going to bed, so as not to interfere with human growth hormone production that occurs when we sleep, stalling weight loss altogether. Any eating outside of this time frame should be limited to drinking water or healthy tea, which is fine. Sleep is also an important part of the equation, with 8 hours being the ideal resting time.

Is a Ketogenic Diet Harmful or Dangerous?

No. There are a lot of misinformation/myths and general 'un-truths' out there on the internet and the public domain about the keto diet. Many people confuse the term '*ketosis*' with the far dangerous state of 'Keto-*acidosis*'. These are two very different conditions. Keto-acidosis is found in Type 1 diabetics that have extremely dangerous levels of low glucose resulting in this state. Ketosis on the other hand is a very natural process of unlocking fats – either in the form of fats we eat or body fats, to fuel the body for metabolic energy. Keto-acidosis therefore would only occur if you were a type 1 diabetic or if you had literally starved for well over a month.

Additionally, the data and actual studies that are formulated are based on incorrect data collated from false criteria from the onset. Often when these clinical studies were initiated they were performed on rodents, mice and rats. The actual "high fat' diet they were fed for the studies was NOT actually a traditional ketogenic diet. Instead what the rodents were fed was a HIGH FAT/HIGH CARB diet – which is NOT a ketogenic diet and YES that would be dangerous. As already explained a keto diet is LOW CARB/HIGH FAT. Specifically, the results from these clinical studies demonstrate the actual macro breakdown to:

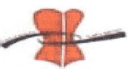

- 24% carbs,
- 21% protein
- And 50% fats.

Comparatively a traditional keto diet is

- 5-10% carbs
- 20 % protein
- And 70-75% fats.

Going further into detail on exactly what type's /categories as well as quality of fats the rodent consumed during the experiment also sheds further light on the myths surrounding keto diets.

The QUALITY of the fats they were fed were indeed dangerous. In fact, 30% of the fat intake was of a 'Trans Fat' category, which as we have already explained in this book thus far, is, indeed highly dangerous and should be AVOIDED. The Ketogenic diet does NOT encourage anyone to consume these in any levels – These are present in processed and manufactured foods.

Next 28% was consumed from the 'saturated fat 'category – which is the animal fats. A ketogenic diet does allow only a moderate-to- low consumption of these. Finally, the Unsaturated fats category – the plant-based fats – including Polyunsaturated and Mon-Unsaturated fats) this category showed the rodents eating LEAST OF– whereas a traditional ketogenic diet favours the unsaturated fats to be MOST consumed.

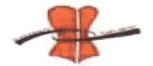

So, you can see the actual studies themselves were incorrectly set up and therefore the result of which do not actually test a ketogenic diet – what these studies do show Is that a diet that is based on manufactured foods, poor quality hydrogenated oils, and high carb intake combined all leads to a dangerous result. This is true!

So instead –when someone does say that a keto diet' is dangerous - ask the source of the clinical study.

I have attached the link to the actual data, so you can check it out yourself.

http://diabetes.diabetesjournals.org/content/diabetes/suppl/2009/08/18/db08-1261.DC1/db08-1261_Online_appendix.pdf

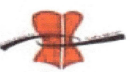

24 Benefits of the Ketogenic Diet

1. Weight Loss

Low Carb, high fat diets have been used for centuries by doctors when working with obese patients. William Banting published the widely popular booklet titled 'Letter on Corpulence Addressed to the Public' in 1863. In this booklet, he explained how he had slimmed down by eating a diet high in fat void of carbs. The Banting diet was used for decades by individuals looking to lose weight.

Though the 'banting' diet may not be a true ketosis diet, it did bring about many traits that are present on a ketogenic diet. One huge benefit being suppressed appetite. Combine this with lowered insulin levels from lack of carbohydrates and you have a 1-2 combination in decreasing body fat levels.

Many people successfully use ketogenic diets today in their quest for decreased body fat levels for these exact reasons. By consuming a higher fat/lower Carb diet, you also retrain the body to use fat as an energy source. This allows the body to tap into its own fat reserves – burning it as energy. If your body is used to burning carbohydrates for fuel, then when those Carb sources run out or are not consumed, your body craves another 'hit' Despite having a plentiful store of fat.

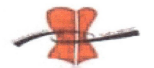

If you are seeking fat loss but do not want to follow a strict ketogenic diet, you will be pleased to know that this study found that the weight loss benefits came purely from a low Carb diet – whether it was ketogenic or not.

2. Anti-aging

Lowering oxidative stress in the body is one way to increase lifespan. It seems that by lowering insulin levels, oxidative stress in turn is decreased. A ketogenic diet decreases insulin levels – allowing the formation of ketones to be used as fuel. Many experts are turning to ketogenic diets in a quest to slow down aging.

3   Lowering Blood Sugar (Type 2 Diabetes)

Speaking of lowered insulin levels, a result of running off ketones allows an individual to control, and lower, their blood sugar levels. The ability to utilise fat and ketones as fuel for the body means a pre-diabetic or even a type 2 diabetic, no longer must worry about excess blood sugar levels and the need to source exogenous insulin.

Bistrian et al documented in the 1976 study how Type 2 Diabetic patients on a ketogenic diet no longer needed insulin and they lost a lot of body weight.

These findings were backed up in a 2012 study which had obese diabetics follow a ketogenic diet for 12 months. The researchers found lower fasting glucose levels, improved cholesterol markers and improved HA1c readings. Remember, carbs and glucose are not required when on a ketogenic diet, as stable, clean burning energy is sourced from fat. This makes controlling blood sugar levels near fool proof.

4.   Cardiovascular Disease and Metabolic Syndrome

If you are still in the belief camp that fat causes cardiovascular disease, you need to read this article -9 Reasons Why Your Doctor is wrong about Fat. In fact, by eating a diet rich in fat and void of carbohydrates, you may be able to reverse cardiovascular disease symptoms.

Research by Dr Jeff Volek & Dr Richard Feinman found that the contributors to heart disease (evaluated blood sugar, high blood triglycerides, low HDL cholesterol, high blood pressure, etc.) are improved when following a low Carb, ketogenic type diet.

5   Polycystic Ovary Syndrome (PCOS)

PCOS often occurs along with insulin resistance – causing a range of hormonal issues in woman – including infertility.

A ketogenic diet – due to its extremely low Carb intake – can help address insulin resistance and in turn help with sufferers of PCOS. In fact, a pilot study has concluded that a ketogenic diet led to a significant improvement in body weight, fasting insulin, testosterone markets and LH/FSH ratio in woman with PCOS. Two women even became pregnant during the study.

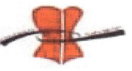

6. Brain Function

Other than fat loss, a big reason why so many people rave about ketogenic diets is due to improved brain function, clarity of thought, memory recall, improved learning, etc.

And science backs up these claims. One study done on rats found that a ketogenic diet leads to cognitive performance in aged rats. Another rat study showed that the ketogenic study was protective against diet induced cognitive impairment (from eating a standard western diet).

A human study found that ketogenic diets, even in the short term, can improve memory function in older adults. Also, a ketogenic diet was shown to increase ATP concentrations and the number of hippocampus* mitochondria in the brain of mice by up to 50%. *The hippocampus is involved in memory, learning and emotion.

Dr Myhill states that the brain (and heart) runs at least 25% more efficiently on ketones than blood sugar. A huge number when you remember that the brain uses up to 20% of the body's total energy.

But the proof is in the pudding, anyone who has experienced a state of ketosis will be able to tell you firsthand the beneficial effects on their cognitive function.

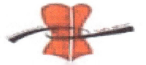

7. Irritable Bowel Syndrome (IBS)

Many who suffer from IBS (chronic diarrhoea, stomach discomfort, bloating etc.) would probably shudder at the thought of eating a high fat low Carb diet. Upping fat intake can lead to increased diarrhoea at first, but it's the long-term effects of a ketogenic diet that are appealing to those suffering from IBS.

Numerous studies have found that low sugar consumption can assist with IBS symptoms and one study found that a ketogenic diet provides adequate relief, and improves abdominal pain, stool habits, and quality of life in individuals suffering from IBS

8. Increased Mitochondrial Function

Mitochondria are our cells' energy factories, without mitochondria in our cells we would be dead. A lot of our health, energy, sports performance, immune function, etc. are dependent upon how well our mitochondria are functioning.

Dr Gabriela Segura explains the connection between a ketogenic diet and increased mitochondria function in the article - Ketogenic Diet: A Connection between Mitochondria and Diet. In that article, she explains how:

"The mitochondria – work much better on a ketogenic diet as they are able to increase energy levels in a stable, long-burning, efficient, and steady way. Not only that, a ketogenic diet induces epigenetic changes [6] which increases the energetic output of our mitochondria, reduces the production of damaging free radicals, and favours the production of GABA".

Mitochondria are specifically designed to use fat for energy. When our mitochondria use fat as an energetic source, its toxic load is decreased, the expression of energy producing genes are increased, its energetic output is increased, and the load of inflammatory energetic-end-products is decreased.

The key of these miraculous healing effects relies on the fact that fat metabolism and its generation of ketone bodies (beta-hydroxybutyrate and acetoacetate) by the liver can only occur within the mitochondrion, leaving chemicals within the cell but outside the mitochondria readily available to stimulate powerful anti-inflammatory antioxidants. The status of our mitochondria is the ultimate key for optimal health, and while it is true that some of us might need extra support in the form of nutritional supplementation to heal these much-needed energy factories, the diet still remains the ultimate key for a proper balance.

9. Endurance Performance

If you are an endurance athlete, and you haven't considered the benefits of ketosis and endurance performance, you are potentially missing out on a massive edge over your competition.

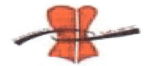

The studies done on ketosis and endurance sports performance paint a clear picture – it helps. One of the most detailed studies on fat utilisation and performance (compared to a standard Carb diet) was named the FASTER study; the results found that those who were on a ketogenic type diet had more mitochondria than the control group, lower oxidative stress, lower lactate load and that the fat adapted, and fuelled athletes could function off fat for a much higher intensity than the non-fat adapted counter parts.

Also, there are numerous studies showing how ketones in the blood lead to significant performance improvements. This paper showed increased power output over a 30-minute period.

A study published in 2016 found supplemental ketone ester supplements "demonstrate that acute nutritional ketosis alters substrate utilization patterns during exercise, reduces lactate production, and improves time-trial performance in elite cyclists."

And Patrick Arnold, creator of the KetoForce supplement, claims that:

"Theoretically, ketones should reduce oxygen consumption because they are known to generate more cellular energy per unit oxygen burned compared to glucose and other energy sources."

All this points towards ketosis (whether it was brought on by dietary changes or supplemental changes) being a potentially huge performance enhancer for endurance athletes.

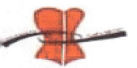

10. Decreased Pain & Lowered Inflammation

Ketosis has been shown to have anti-inflammatory properties while also assisting with pain relief. Reducing glucose metabolism influences pain, so this could be one potential mechanism of action. In the review, The Nervous System and Metabolic Deregulation: Emerging Evidence Converges on Ketogenic Diet Therapy, the authors look at numerous ways that a ketogenic diet can assist with pain and inflammation.

11. Stable Energy Levels

Anyone who has recently switched from a standard western diet to a ketogenic diet will soon notice how their energy levels are stable throughout the day. No mid-afternoon slumps, no cravings for instant sugar or caffeine hits.

Fat (and the ketones produced from fat) are a readily available source of fuel. Once someone is fat adapted and in ketosis, they will find they can easily go hours (even days) without food and not have drastic energy level swings.

12. Heartburn

A study published in the Journal of Digestive Diseases and Sciences found that after less than a week on a ketogenic diet, study participants with GERD (Gastroesophageal reflux disease) all showed a reduction in acidity in the oesophagus (linked to heart burn) and the participants reported less severity in their heart burn conditions. All this achieved simply from removing carbohydrates from the diet and increasing the fat intake.

13. Fatty Liver Disease

As per heartburn, studies done have shown that a ketogenic diet can have beneficial effects for those who have Non-Alcoholic Fatty Liver Disease. A 2006 paper published in the Journal of Digestive Diseases and Sciences found that 'Six months of a low-carbohydrate, ketogenic diet led to significant weight loss and histological improvement of fatty liver disease'. This was only a pilot study with 5 individuals, but there have been bigger studies done since the 2006 paper that support its findings.

14. Migraine Treatment

Many people who suffer from migraines have reported great results when switching from a conventional high Carb diet to an ultra-low Carb ketogenic diet. But it's not just anecdotal evidence that shows the beneficial connection between ketosis and migraine treatment; a study published in the Journal of Headache Pain concluded:

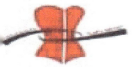

Ketogenic diets (KD) ameliorates headache and reduces drug consumption in migraineurs, while the Standard diet is fully ineffective on migraine in a short-term observation. Our findings support the role of KDs in migraine treatment.

Another paper looked at twin sisters who suffered from frequent migraines, but when switched to a ketogenic diet, the frequency and severity of their migraines decreased.

15. Clean Burning Fuel for the Body

There is a reason why we store hundreds of thousands of calories in the form of fat in our body and only about 2000 calories in the form of glucose (with only a small amount of this useable by the brain). The reason is simple - The body prefers fat as its fuel source. Mark Sisson explains this in his article, 'A metabolic Paradigm Shift or Why Fat is the Preferred Fuel for Human Consumption'.

When cells break down glucose for fuel, they generate more reactive oxygen species compared to fat. These free radicals are neutralised by antioxidants. So, skip the supplements, restrict carbohydrates, eat more fat and operate off clean burning ketones instead!

16. Mood Stabilisation (Autism & Bipolar etc.)

A quick Google search of autism + ketosis will bring up 100s of articles where people share their tales of improving autism with a ketogenic diet. Why? Because it appears that ketosis is extremely effective for dealing with autism.

The research paper, Potential Therapeutic Use of the Ketogenic Diet in Autism Spectrum Disorders, remarked that ketogenic diets were seen to be beneficial when it came to be dealing with autism, but that more research was needed.

One study was done on 30 Autistic children; the ketogenic diet – with 30% of MCT oil – was administered for 6 months. The children with the milder autistic behaviours showed the most improvement, while the rest displayed mild to moderate improvements.

A fascinating find from this study was that the beneficial effects of the ketogenic diet continued even after the trial ended. There are also numerous reports of ketosis helping with mood stabilization in individuals suffering from bipolar.

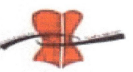

17. Easier to Fast

One of the best ways to get into a state of ketosis is through fasting. However, anyone who is eating a standard high Carb diet will shudder at the thought of going 12 hours or longer without food.

Yet once you are fat adapted and you are in a state of nutritional ketosis, fasting becomes extremely easy.

18. Parkinson's Disease

Ketosis has also been shown to help those suffering from Parkinson's disease. 5 individuals suffering from Parkinson's disease followed a ketogenic diet for 28 days, after the 4-week period, all reported improved ratings in the unified Parkinson's disease rating scale

19. Epilepsy

The ketogenic diet has long been successfully used with those suffering from epilepsy. In fact, the ketogenic diet was first developed in 1921 to treat drug resistant epilepsy in children. Since then, numerous studies have been done showing how ketosis can help with epilepsy. Like the autism study listed above, there is even evidence that epileptic children continued to be seizure free long after they stopped their ketogenic trials.

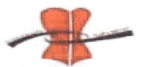

20. Alzheimer's

A lot of scientists are starting to believe that Alzheimer's should be considered 'type 3' diabetes – as the brain becomes unable to utilise glucose (insulin resistant) leading to high levels of inflammation. If the brain cannot utilise glucose, and we know that under the right circumstances the brain can operate off ketones, then it would lead you to believe that a ketogenic diet may assist with Alzheimer's. There are now studies being published that support this link. One paper concluded that "a significant clinical improvement was observed in Alzheimer's patients fed a ketogenic diet".

And there are more research studies that support the beneficial link between ketosis and Alzheimer's.

21. Cancer

Ketosis as a form of cancer treatment (and prevention) is rapidly growing in popularity. Why is that? It is because so many cancer patients are reporting huge benefits when following a ketogenic diet. And why may that be? Many cancer cells can only survive with glucose as a fuel source.

By depriving a cancer cell of glucose by eating a ketogenic diet, we may be able to starve the cancer resulting in its death.

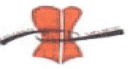

If you're thinking this all sounds too good to be true, then you may want to check out this paper – 'Is there a role for carbohydrate restriction in the treatment and prevention of cancer?' In this book: Cancer as a Metabolic Disease' -Seyfried expands upon Otto Warburg's theory that all cancer is a disease of energy metabolism.

And science is now catching up, this review paper on ketogenic diets as a form of cancer therapy concluded: "Although the mechanism by which ketogenic diets demonstrate anticancer effects … has not been fully elucidated, preclinical results have demonstrated the safety and potential efficacy of using ketogenic diets. Improve responses in murine cancer models".

While a mouse study found that ketone supplementation decreased tumour cell viability and extended survival rates in mice with cancer.

Finally, a feasibility study was done on 10 cancer patients in 2012. All patients followed a ketogenic diet for 28 days after exhausting every other cancer treatment option. The results of the study found that 1 had a partial remission of their cancer, 5 stabilized and 4 continued progressing. It's important to remember that these individuals had tried all other forms of cancer treatment. 60% of these individuals then stalled or improved their cancer rates by following a ketogenic diet for 4 weeks.

22. Multiple Sclerosis (MS)

Perhaps the biggest anecdotal evidence on ketosis slowing down MS is the story of Dr Terry Wahl's. Dr Wahl's overcame being wheelchair bound after trying various drugs and conventional therapies without success. Eventually, she turned to dietary changes – including following a ketogenic diet – and a lot of her symptoms disappeared. She now lives an active life, riding horses and going on long treks. She shares her story and the protocol she developed in the book, 'The Wahl's Protocol: A Radical New Way to Treat All Chronic Autoimmune Conditions Using Paleo Principles'.

Dr Wahl's is leading the charge into MS treatment using a ketogenic diet, but until some of her studies are published, we can look at mice studies that also show the benefits of ketosis with mice with MS.

23. Acne

There is a lot of emerging evidence that ketosis can help clear acne. It has been shown that high glycolic foods can stimulate acne outbreaks, and as the ketogenic diet goes without such foods, it makes sense that acne should improve.

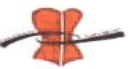

Some studies have shown a positive connection between ketosis and lower levels of ketosis, but as Paoli et all conclude in their paper, Beyond Weight Loss: a review of the therapeutic uses of very-low-carbohydrate (ketogenic) diets, there is persuasive, although not yet conclusive, clinical and physiological evidence that the ketogenic diet could be effective in reducing the severity and progression of acne and randomized clinical trials will be required to resolve the issue.

24. General Health and Well-being

We have already looked at the links between ketosis and diseases like cancer, Alzheimer's, epilepsy and fatty liver disease, amongst others. But studies have also shown that following a ketogenic diet lead to:

- Improved cholesterol levels
- Decreased triglyceride levels
- Decreased weight and fat mass
- Not to mention the countless other benefits shared online

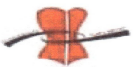

Chapter 7: How to get started with Keto

OK, so we have covered a lot so far. Let's re-cap:

We have looked at:

The reasons why we gain and have difficulty losing fat, particularly in those stubborn areas.

Which hormones have an effect on whether we hold onto fat or burn fat? These are all run by the endocrine system in our body and the main culprits for weight are:

- Insulin
- Insulin resistance
- Cortisol
- Estrogen

Mindset is a big part of weight loss- How we think and what we say to ourselves in our mind has a huge effect on how we feel about ourselves and the actions we take or don't take in life that consequently give us the results we have now.

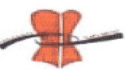

Goal setting – Clearly state what you want to achieve. Choose your 'WHY'. Losing weight is NOT easy – even if so many weight loss programs will tell you it is – its hard work – so you need to have the right MINDSET and know why you are doing this. I imagine it will be because of the love of your children, family and ultimately yourself and for general health and well-being.

Choosing the right types of foods particularly those that are natural fat burners as well as having additional health benefits. By merely substituting some ingredients you currently eat, with these, you will be making small but consistent steps forward to your end goal.

Detoxing – You will need to detox away from high sugar processed and manufactured foods. Start looking for REAL foods instead of something that comes out of a box from a factory. Get back to basics. Strip away all the inflammatory food. Start to 'listen' to your body. If something gives you pain, indigestion, excessive wind, acne, etc., it means it's inflammatory to your body. Listen to your body's signs and either eliminate those foods or substitute for something healthier.

7-day meal plan – This is a low calorie standard meal plan to lose weight. Results following this plan vary from person to person.

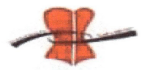

Finally, we moved into an introduction of the ketogenic diet, what is involved and what are the multiple benefits of following such a diet and what are the myths.

Overall, the main aim is to get you healthy, and once your body is healthy and all your hormones are balanced and working properly, you WILL naturally lose the body fat. The weight is just a symptom that your body is not healthy.

So, in this chapter, let me tell you how to transition into a keto diet which will OPTIMISE your fat loss and literally melt that fat away that you have been trying so hard to get rid of.

Transitioning into Keto for Weight Loss

As we have covered previously, the body traditionally uses glucose (or carbohydrates) as its main source of energy. However, there is another source which the body can use and that is through fats. Now, fats can come in 2 forms, either:

1. Fats that we eat
2. Or stored body fats

It is through the liver and mitochondria that ketone bodies will break down fats so that it can be used as an alternative source of metabolic energy to fuel its needs.

Now, up until now – reading this book, you have always been told that the only way to burn fat and lose weight is to cut calories and go into a calorie deficit. – Basically, starving yourself of your body's nutritional needs. Now, don't get me wrong, being in a calorie deficit is helpful short term and in itself is a metabolic state of ketosis– however, it's the nutrients and the macro-components the QUALITY that makes up those calories that we are going to focus on with keto.

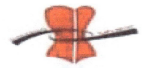

First step you would have already taken back in the chapters 4 & 5 with the carb detox. This is an important stage as the body cannot use 2 different types of fuel at the same time. It will either favour one or the other. So, we need to shift over and transition away from a diet that is high in carbohydrates. Now, for clarity, carbohydrates include:

- Complex carbohydrates
- Simple Carbohydrates

Many of us know the complex carbohydrates - our breads, pastas, rice, oats, wheat, grains, etc.

Simple carbohydrates are fruits and vegetables. So, you need to be conscious of the simple carbohydrates you eat as well as those 'hidden' carbs that are found in products, sauces, dressings, etc.

Even dairy can be high in carbohydrates particularly yoghurts, so watch these! Many people often discover they are intolerant of dairy and find it is a cause of inflammation.

Keep fruits low but eat lots of vegetables.

You will be getting all your macro carbohydrates from the vegetables as well as your micro-nutrients - all the essential vitamins and minerals that your body needs. So, eat as much vegetables as you like. Limit fruit and AVOID starchy carbs.

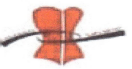

When you move into keto, your macro breakdown is going to look like this:

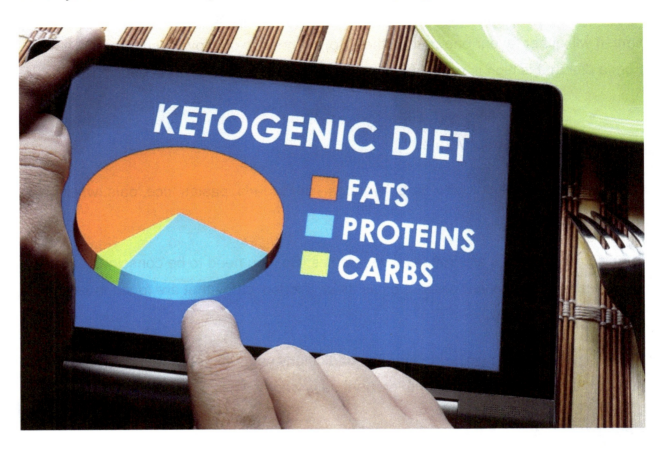

Now, most people usually freak out when they initially hear the high fat component. So please, before you do that, give yourself a chance to understand the process through this book and my videos - how the body works and why this is such an effective way of losing weight as well as fuelling the body with everything it needs.

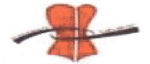

I admit it does seem odd, as it did for me, that by eating fat you can lose weight. It sounds kind of counter-intuitive. A lot of it comes down to the way we have always been educated on food and nutrition. Even from school age with the food pyramid telling us to eat breads and cereals the most and fats the least.

Yet millions of people around the world are suffering from obesity and it's growing bigger into epidemic proportions. Weight related diseases are at an all-time high that could be prevented with proper health and nutrition.

To help you understand a little more about why the keto diet is so effective, I am going to explain more about what fats do in the body, why you need them, which ones to eat, and which to avoid:

Along with protein, fats have an essential function in the body.

- ✓ Fats are essential as they give you energy.
- ✓ Keep your body warm.
- ✓ They build your cells.
- ✓ Protect your organs.
- ✓ Help your body absorb essential vitamins and minerals from your food.
- ✓ And they produce the hormones that your body needs to work properly.

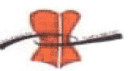

Getting down to basics, there are 3 categories when it comes to dietary fats.

1. Trans-fats
2. Saturated fats
3. Unsaturated fats

The difference between these three (3) types of fats lies in their chemical composition. All fats are made up of carbon atoms that are linked or bonded to a hydrogen atom.

Trans Fats

Trans Fats are the manufactured fats that have gone through a process called 'hydrogenation'. You'll probably see these listed on your ingredients labelled as 'partly - hydrogenated oils' to disguise the fact that these are actually Trans Fats.

Trans Fats are created to make foods:

- Last longer on the shelf/supermarket
- Improve the taste
- Improve the texture

You'll find trans-fat in cakes, pies, cookies, biscuits, crackers, margarine, etc. All those yummy things – right!

But whilst Trans Fats may taste good – they are **NOT good** for you!!

AVOID Trans Fats at all costs!

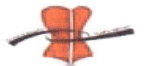

Saturated Fats

Saturated fats are where the carbon atoms are completely covered with a hydrogen atom or "saturated", and this is also what makes them solid at room temperature.

Saturated fats are basically your animal fats like cheese, butter, yoghurt, cream, eggs and coconut oil, feel free to eat these in MODERATION.

Unsaturated Fats

Unsaturated fats have fewer carbon atoms that are boded and hence liquid at room temperature.

These are the Fats that I want you to **EAT MOST OF.** These are mainly plant-based fats. These are broken down into 2 more types:

1. Monounsaturated
2. Polyunsaturated

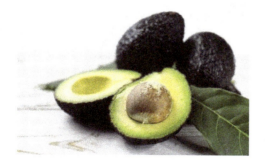

Monounsaturated Fats

'Mono' meaning one, has one chemical bond attached. These are your avocados, olive oils, peanut oils, nuts: almonds, hazelnuts and macadamias.

Polyunsaturated fats

Poly' – meaning many chemical bonds attached. These are your 'Essential Fatty Acids'. (EFA) Flaxseeds, walnuts, leafy green vegetables, fatty fish, salmon tuna, mackerel, and sardines.

These are going to give you your **Omega 3 and Omega 6s**.

Your **heart and your brain absolutely LOVE these.**

So, to sum up: when it comes to the ketogenic diet, you're going to be:

1. Reducing your carbohydrates low - focusing mainly on small amount of fruit= as this contains sugar but eats lots of vegetables. (7-10 cups per day)

2. A moderate amount of protein – stick with the guidelines of 0.8g per Kg of body weight as a guide. Don't overeat protein as this can lead to being converted to glucose and stored as fat. It also puts a lot of pressure on the liver.

3. And high fats. The fats you choose will be the polyunsaturated fats and unsaturated fats. (Moderate animal fats/more nuts/avocados/salmon etc.)

Remember your fats can also come from stored body fats so you don't have to eat it all from your diet – you will be accessing your stored fat that's sitting on your belly, hips, thighs and wherever …. Via ketones (endogenous/exogenous ketones) – which I will share in the next chapter….

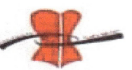

Chapter 8: Ketones

What are Ketones?

Ketones exist in every healthy human being inside our blood cells. They are produced by the liver and allow our body to convert fat into a useable source of metabolic energy. They are an alternative fuel source to glucose. Ketones are simple compounds because of their small molecular structure and weight. Specifically, they are organic (carbon-based) compounds that contain a central carbon atom double-bonded to an oxygen atom and two carbon-containing substituents, denoted by "R" (see chemical structure below).

In our bodies, there are 3 different ketones produced by the mitochondria of the liver. Think of the mitochondria as the 'power factory' of your cells. Their job is to convert calories from food, heat from the sun and oxygen into energy and keep your blood pumping. So, these ketones are going to increase what's known as 'Mitochondrial biogenesis. What that means is that it will increase the number of mitochondria in your cells. Therefore, having more power factories available in your body to help spread the workload is ultimately going to help your body work more efficiently.

If we look more closely at the chemical composition of these ketones (also known as 'ketone bodies') we know that there are three different types:

I'm Sick of Being Fat! – Sarah Jane

1. Acetoacetate (or also known as Acetoacetic Acid
2. Acetone
3. Beta-Hydroxybutyric Acid (also known Beta Hydroxybutyrate or BHB).

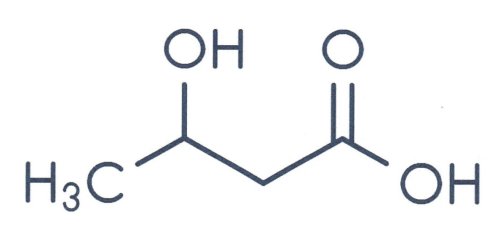

Acetoacetate is the 'mother molecule' here, and when the body is triggered into a state of ketosis (by being depleted of glucose in the blood) it then breaks down into 2 more molecules. Those two molecules are as listed above: Acetone and Beta Hydroxybutyrate (BHB). The Acetone moves on to get utilised elsewhere in the cells and the BHB helps to 'unlock' the fat cells to release the fat back into the mitochondria, into the blood stream and around the body and the brain to be utilised as the reserve source of energy.

To put all this chemistry, simply, think of Beta Hydroxybutyrate as the 'storage molecule'. A little bit like in your home when you have a lot of excess food left over from the week or a meal. You don't want to waste the food, so you would take the excess food and place it into the freezer, that way you could use it later, when you really needed it. Similarly, this is what happens in the body.

It is a very natural process that humans have been using for hundreds of years. Particularly during a period of famine. This process allowed us to get through these times, allowing our bodies to utilise our stored body fats as a source of energy until our next meal was available.

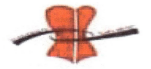

So, these ketone bodies are a 'key' to unlocking energy efficiently. Without these ketones, we would literally die during any fasting, as the brain can only function on glucose. (This is why it was so commonly thought that we needed carbohydrates in our diet). These ketones, thus can convert via these compounds, send it to the mitochondria in the cells and thus pass through the blood-brain barrier.

As discussed in the previous chapter, the benefits of ketones are obvious; however, for many of us sticking to a strict ketogenic diet is very difficult so the question remains – what is the best way to increase your ketone levels?

Exogenous Ketones

What are they and How Can They Help You?

The concept of a ketogenic diet may be simple to grasp, however, getting into a state of ketosis and maintaining ketosis and a ketogenic can prove challenging. Fortunately, we now have access to 'Exogenous ketones'. Exogenous ketones have become a very popular nutritional supplement since their introduction in 2014. They have been brought into the limelight when the US Navy Seals contracted Professor Dom D'Agostino. The Office of Navy Research funded Dom D'Agostino's project to investigate these ketones specifically for performance enhancement, physical performance and cognitive performance for their Navy SEAL Fighters

His research and studies led to laboratory testing to create an artificial ketone body that would literally 'mimic' the exact same effects and benefits of endogenous ketone bodies without the need to stick to a strict ketogenic diet. Studies are even finding that supplementation with exogenous ketones is superior to the ketogenic diet. Even while following a Standard North American Diet (SAD), individuals can still experience the benefits of ketones via supplementation. However, it is thought that following a lower carbohydrate diet, not necessarily a strict ketogenic diet, will enhance the benefits of the ketone supplements, as your body becomes even more adept to using the ketones as a source of fuel.

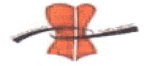

There are two methods the body can source the ketone bodies:

- **Exogenous** - Originates from a source external from the body. E.g. orally via a supplement.
- **Endogenous** - Originates from a source internal to the body – produced in the liver, i.e., following the traditional ketogenic diet – (Low Carbs/ Medium Protein and High Fats)

So, exogenous ketone bodies are just ketone bodies that are ingested through a nutritional supplement. Ketone bodies produced in the liver are more properly referred to as endogenous ketone bodies.

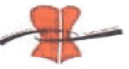

What are the Benefits of Exogenous Ketones?

Exogenous ketone supplements may provide a multitude of benefits.

These include:

- Athletic performance enhancement.
- More efficient weight loss.
- Cancer prevention.
- Cognitive improvement.
- Anti-inflammatory properties.

So How Will Exogenous Ketones help me to Burn More Fat?

Appetite Control:

Because your brain is getting a supply of high powered energy in the form of ketones, it reduces the demand for further calories from food. A recent study at the University of Melbourne published in the European Journal of Clinical Nutrition showed that when overweight subjects were placed on a calorie restricted ketogenic diet, they lost 13% of their bodyweight. The subjects experienced no increase in Ghrelin (the appetite increasing hormone) that is normally seen with calorie restricted diets. The participants subjectively had a lower perceived appetite than those on a non-ketogenic calorie restricted diet. Therefore, Ketones may keep hunger pangs away by controlling Ghrelin and improving Leptin (appetite controlling hormone) sensitivity.

Mitochondrial Biogenesis:

There are several ways ketones work to burn body fat. The most important is its ability to increase mitochondrial biogenesis (the number of mitochondria). As described earlier, mitochondria are like the fat burning power engines of your cells. Often genetically gifted athletes or people that are naturally lean have higher amounts of mitochondria per cell. Therefore, they burn fat faster and provide thus more energy to their body. If you can increase the number and efficiency of your mitochondria, it stands to reason that you will also become more efficient at burning fat, especially with the addition of Acetyl L-Carnitine.

Blood Sugar Metabolism:

Ketosis or the supplementation of exogenous ketones may help to improve insulin sensitivity which may result in your body utilizing carbohydrates (sugars) more efficiently. If you use carbs more efficiently, you are less likely to store them as body fat.

How do Ketones Assist with Brain Function?

Improved cognition:

Elevated plasma ketone concentrations divert the brain to utilize ketone bodies for synthesis of phospholipids, which drives growth and myelination. Normally, glucose would be the preferred substrate, which is much less efficient. Ketones are arguably the preferred source of energy for our brains and we can use them very efficiently. There are multiple mechanisms involved in the mental improvements seen in ketogenic subjects, including a reduction in the mental decline of those suffering from Alzheimer's, Dementia and Parkinson's. Much of these benefits may be due to the improved blood sugar management seen with ketones

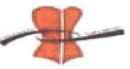

Improved mood:

Other benefits may include improved brain mitochondrial function, reduced inflammation and increased BDNF (Brain Derived Neurotrophic Factor). BDNF is a naturally occurring hormone that protects and repairs your brain cells, increases the growth of new brain cells, and improves learning, memory and mood. In fact, many researchers consider it a natural antidepressant. Research suggests that if you struggle with mental illness, brain fog or poor brain function, you likely have reduced levels of BDNF. Ketones may help to enhance the production of BDNF. On every 1.0 m/mol of ketones in the blood, there is approximately a 10% improvement in brain function.

What about my Performance Goals?

Athletic enhancement:

Exogenous ketone supplementation has a promising outlook for enhancing athletic performance for a variety of reasons. Firstly, ingested ketone bodies induce an acute ketosis that lasts for several hours and mimics the physiology of starvation.

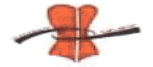

Secondly, exogenous ketones present a way to elevate ketone levels without having depleted muscle glycogen stores (low muscle glycogen is well known to impair sustained physical performance). Currently, there is little direct data that shows performance enhancements after ingesting exogenous ketones. A very well formulated study by Volek et al. has shown that fat adapted athletes have much higher glycogen stores than was previously anticipated and the athletes can replenish glycogen stores as efficiently as athletes on a carbohydrate-based diet. The hypothetical premise behind their use is sound nevertheless.

What about Health & Longevity?

Anti-carcinogenic properties:

Data seems to suggest that exogenous ketones are an effective anti-carcinogen. The reason behind this is that cancer cells are unable to use ketone bodies effectively, unlike most healthy tissues in the body. In fact, dietary ketone supplementation has been shown to increase survival rates of mice with systematic cancer by as much as 70%. That must be exciting news for you or anyone you love who is touched by cancer.

Neuroprotection:

As humans age, the brain becomes more susceptible to neurodegeneration and subsequent conditions such as Alzheimer's and Parkinson's disease. Exogenous ketone supplementation appears to ameliorate the typical decline in cognitive function that comes with aging. The likely mechanism for this neuroprotective property is that ketone bodies reduce the inflammation and hyperexcitability that is normally exhibited as glucose metabolism declines in the brain.

Anti-Inflammatory properties: There is evidence that ketone bodies play a crucial role in reducing inflammation by inhibiting a specific class of proteins called inflammasomes

Ok-So, how do I Get These Exogenous Ketone Supplements?

There are many different manufacturers of exogenous ketone supplements. I will let you know my experiences and will leave it up to try and test if you wish or save your money and get the best.

When I first heard about exogenous ketones – I was so excited! Not having to be careful about macro nutrients on the keto diet was a plus together with these incredible benefits that were previously described.

Initially, they were ONLY available in the US. This meant that I had to import the product from overseas; a currency exchange rate added more costs plus the international shipping at US rates. Then I had to wait approximately 2 months before I even got it.

I tried a few brands, there is an MLM organisation – some people feel empowered to be a part of this, although it wasn't my cup of tea. What I noticed by reading the ingredients and quantities is there seemed to be a lot of variance in the levels of BHB listed. What I was really aiming for was MAXIMUM VALUE for MONEY.

I wanted all the benefits promised and above and beyond - TASTE was extremely important to me. So, after trialling and testing numerous products, there was one product that shone head and shoulders above the rest. It ticked all the boxes for me………..

My Special Thank You to You for Reading This Book….

Introducing

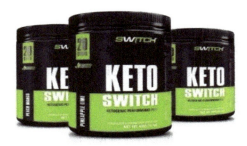

As a special thank you for reading my book, I am going to offer you….

10% OFF the R.R.P!

The one supplement that GUARANTEES to put you into ketosis within 30 MINUTES! https://switchnutrition.com.au/discount/SARAH10

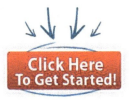

Continue with Your Journey

Well, my friend we have completed your introduction to the keto lifestyle. I am **certain** that if you have read every single page of this book and tried everything I suggested, you would undoubtedly have already noticed a change in your body, health and life. That dream you started with when you first picked up this book, of losing that extra stubborn fat, is no longer a dream, it is reality. But as the Carpenters sang, 'We've only just begun!'

You have learnt in detail how your body functions in relation to weight gain. Hopefully, you have now got an understanding of the relevant hormones involved in storage and burning of fats as well as what controls the appetite. The key is in controlling these hormones with the help of the right nutrition, to help you achieve the results you desire. Follow a healthy ketogenic diet and use your exogenous ketone supplements to support you along the way, to speed up as well as enhance your results. Set your goals strong. Keep going and strive higher and higher.

You may also be excited by the changes or new possibilities but really need that extra support. You may need someone to hold you by the hand and go through step-by-step exactly what to do. Maybe identify which hormones are imbalanced and get more personal assistance. If that's you then I do offer an exclusive online members program that does all this for you.

Go to: http://www.ketowithsarahjane.com

Lots of love and support always!

Your friend,

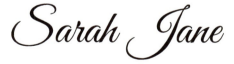

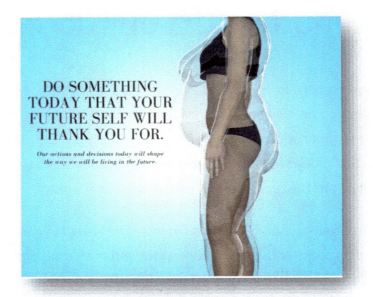

Follow us on our community-based Facebook following – find people just like you in their journey to heath and bettering themselves.

https://www.facebook.com/ketowithsarahjane/

For lots of educational videos on the keto lifestyle, recipes, science, interviews and more, subscribe to: keto with Sarah jane

https://www.youtube.com/channel/UCIr-ULOgqs_w3iLwx6Fd4BA

Need that extra help to really get this implemented and working for you?

Join our exclusive members only online program.

Go to http://www.ketowithsarahjane.com

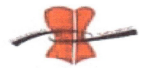

References:

- Articles
- Bianco A, Canato M, Fratter A, Grimaldi K, Paoli A, Toniolo L, Therapeutic Potential of Ketogenic Diets" (2012)
- Julie Corliss, 5 Habits that Foster Weight Loss", (2017) Harvard Health Publications, Harvard Medical School
- Cox, P. J, & Clarke, K (2014). <u>Acute nutritional ketosis: implications for exercise performance and metabolism.</u> Extreme Physiology & Medicine, 3, 17.
- D'Agostino, D. P., Pilla, R., Held, H. E., Landon, C. S., Puchowicz, M., Brunengraber, H., & Dean, J. B. (2013). Therapeutic ketosis with ketone ester delays central nervous system oxygen toxicity seizures in rats. American Journal of Physiology-Regulatory, Integrative and Comparative Physiology, 304(10), R829-R836.
- Hashim, S. A., & VanItallie, T. B. (2014). Ketone body therapy: from the ketogenic diet to the oral administration of ketone ester. Journal of lipid research, 55(9), 1818-1826.
- Hertz, L., Chen, Y., & Waagepetersen, H. S. (2015). "Effects of ketone bodies in Alzheimer's disease in relation to neural hypometabolism, β-amyloid toxicity, and astrocyte function". Journal of neurochemistry, 134(1), 7-20.
- Hoffer LJ, Bistrian BR, Young VR, Blackburn GL, Matthews DE "Nutrition and Acne:
- Jorge Bacallao Manuel Pena "Obesity and Poverty: A New Public Health Challenge" (2000), Pan American Health Organization
- Panda S, Kar A. Changes in thyroid hormone concentrations after administration of ashwaganda root extract to adult male mice. Journal of Pharmacology 1998, 50:1065-1068.
- Poff, A. M., Ari, C., Arnold, P., Seyfried, T. N., & D'Agostino, D. P. (2014). Ketone supplementation decreases tumor cell viability and prolongs survival of mice with metastatic cancer. International journal of cancer, 135 (7), 1711-1720

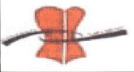

- *Shannon L. Kesl, corresponding author Angela M. Poff, Nathan P. Ward, Tina N. Fiorelli, Csilla Ari, Ashley J. Van Putten, Jacob W. Sherwood, Patrick Arnold, and Dominic P. D'Agostino' <u>Effects of exogenous ketone supplementation on blood ketone, glucose, triglyceride, and lipoprotein levels in Sprague –Dawley rats.</u> (2016 "Nutrition & Metabolism" 13(9*

- *Volek, J. Freidenreich, D.J. Saenz, C. Kunces, L.J. Creighton, B.C. Bartley, J.M. Davitt, P.M. Munoz, C.X. Anderson, J.M. Maresh, C.M. Lee, C.E. Schuenke, M.D. Aemi. G. Kraemer, W.J. Phinney, S.J. (2016)." <u>Metabolic characteristics of keto-adapted ultra-endurance athletes.</u>" 65(3), 100-110.*

- *Yeh, Y. Y., & Sheehan, P. M. "<u>Preferential utilization of ketone bodies in the brain and lung of newborn rats</u>' (1985, April) In Federation proceedings (Vol. 44, No. 7, pp. 2352-2358).*

- *Youm, Y. H., Nguyen, K. Y., Grant, R. W., Goldberg, E. L., Bodogai, M., Kim, D., ... & Kang, S. (2015).<u>The ketone metabolite [beta]-hydroxybutyrate blocks NLRP3 inflammasome-mediated inflammatory disease.</u> Nature medicine, 21(3), 263-269.*

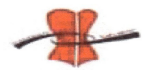

Journals

- *"The Global Strategy on Diet, Physical Activity and Health"* (2008), World Health Organization
- *"Choosing a Safe and Successful Weight-loss Program"* (2012), National Institute of Health, U.S. Department of Health and Human Services
- *"Does Metabolism Matter in Weight Loss?"* (2015), Harvard Health Publications, Harvard Medical School
- *"Healthy Eating After 50"* (2015), National Institute of Health, U.S. Department of Health and Human Services
- *"Metabolic Effects of Very Low-Calorie Weight Reduction Diets"* (1984) J Clin Invest

1. Websites
2. http://www.mirror.co.uk/all-about/weight-loss-success-
3. http://www.womenshealthandfitness.com.au/weight-loss/fat-loss/1652-5-hormones-that-cause-weight-gain
4. https://iquitsugar.com/stages-of-sugar-withdrawal-symptoms/
5. https://authoritynutrition.com/coffee-increase-metabolism/
6. http://health.usnews.com/wellness/articles/2016-09-19/10-ways-to-shift-your-mindset-for-better-weight-loss
7. https://switchnutrition.com.au/products/keto-switch-bhb-ketones
8. https://switchnutrition.com.au/discount/SARAH10
9. http://www.mensfitnessmagazine.com.au/2017/06/the-supp-revolution/
10. https://www.alexfergus.com/blog/24-benefits-of-the-ketogenic-diet
11. https://www.ruled.me/ketosis-ketones-and-how-it-works/
12. https://ketosource.co.uk/exogenous-ketones-how-they-work/

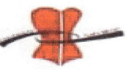

Images

1. Shutter stock
2. I-stock
3. Getty images
4. Switch Nutrition images c/o company director – Greg Haglund
5. Personal photographs supplied by Sarah Jane

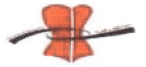

CPSIA information can be obtained
at www.ICGtesting.com
Printed in the USA
LVHW061118311022
731984LV00011B/267